PARTNERS IN HEALTH

PARTNERS IN HEALTH

How Physicians and Hospitals Can Be Accountable Together

Francis J. Crosson

Laura A. Tollen

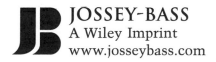

JOSSEY-BASS
A Wiley Imprint
www.josseybass.com

Published by Jossey-Bass
A Wiley Imprint
989 Market Street, San Francisco, CA 94103-1741—www.josseybass.com

Readers should be aware that Internet Web sites offered as citations and/or sources for further information may have changed or disappeared between the time this was written and when it is read.

Limit of Liability/Disclaimer of Warranty: While the publisher and author have used their best efforts in preparing this book, they make no representations or warranties with respect to the accuracy or completeness of the contents of this book and specifically disclaim any implied warranties of merchantability or fitness for a particular purpose. No warranty may be created or extended by sales representatives or written sales materials. The advice and strategies contained herein may not be suitable for your situation. You should consult with a professional where appropriate. Neither the publisher nor author shall be liable for any loss of profit or any other commercial damages, including but not limited to special, incidental, consequential, or other damages.

Jossey-Bass books and products are available through most bookstores. To contact Jossey-Bass directly call our Customer Care Department within the U.S. at 800-956-7739, outside the U.S. at 317-572-3986, or fax 317-572-4002.

Jossey-Bass also publishes its books in a variety of electronic formats. Some content that appears in print may not be available in electronic books.

Library of Congress Cataloging-in-Publication Data

Partners in health : how physicians and hospitals can be accountable together / [edited by] Francis J. Crosson, Laura A. Tollen.—1st ed.
      p. ; cm.
   Includes bibliographical references and index.
   ISBN 978-0-470-55096-0 (cloth)
   1. Hospital-physician joint ventures—United States.   I. Crosson, Francis J., 1945-   II. Tollen, Laura A.
   [DNLM: 1. Delivery of Health Care, Integrated—United States.   2. Health Care Reform—United States.   3. Hospital-Physician Relations—United States. W 84 AA1 P273 2010]
   RA410.58.P37 2010
   362.11068—dc22

                                                                          2010003890

Printed in the United States of America
FIRST EDITION
HB Printing 10 9 8 7 6 5 4 3 2 1

CONTENTS

FIGURES AND TABLES

Figures

Tables

ACKNOWLEDGMENTS

The editors gratefully acknowledge the support of the Kaiser Permanente Institute for Health Policy and the Council of Accountable Physician Practices. We are especially indebted to Murray Ross and Nancy Taylor.

We also wish to acknowledge those who advised us early in the development of this book and helped to identify key topics and authors: Bob Berenson of the Urban Institute, John Iglehart of *Health Affairs,* Mark Miller of MedPAC, Sara Singer of the Harvard School of Public Health, Patricia Smith of the Alliance of Community Health Plans, and Nick Wolter of the Billings Clinic. The fine team at Booz Allen Hamilton, led by Kristine Martin Anderson, was also invaluable in the development and management of this work.

Finally, we want to thank our authors, who contributed their time and expertise, not just in writing their own chapters but in providing input and advice to one another and to the editors, so that the whole of this work is truly more than the sum of its parts.

To all those in America who lack access to affordable, high-quality health care.

THE EDITORS

Francis J. Crosson, MD, is senior fellow of the Kaiser Permanente Institute for Health Policy and associate executive director of the Permanente Medical Group. He has had a career of more than thirty years with Kaiser Permanente, including ten years as executive director of the Permanente Federation, the physician side of that organization. He founded and continues to chair the Council of Accountable Physician Practices. He also serves as vice chairman of the Medicare Payment Advisory Commission, the federal panel that advises the U.S. Congress on Medicare issues.

Laura A. Tollen, MPH, is senior policy consultant at the Kaiser Permanente Institute for Health Policy. Her work focuses on the potential of organized health care delivery systems to contain costs and improve the quality and safety of care. Prior to joining Kaiser Permanente, she was project director at the Institute for Health Policy Solutions, an independent policy think tank. She holds a bachelor's and an MPH, both from the University of California, Berkeley. She is the author of numerous journal articles and the coeditor, with Alain Enthoven, of *Toward a 21st Century Health System: The Contributions and Promise of Prepaid Group Practice.* (Jossey-Bass, 2004).

THE CONTRIBUTORS

Jeffrey A. Alexander, PhD, is Richard C. Jelinek Professor of Health Management and Policy at the University of Michigan School of Public Health. His teaching and research interests focus on organizational change in the health care sector, multi-institutional systems, and policymaking. His recent articles have appeared in *Health Services Research, Milbank Quarterly, Medical Care Research and Review, Administrative Science Quarterly,* and *Journal of Health and Social Behavior.*

Lawton R. Burns, PhD, MBA, is professor of health care management and director at the Wharton Center for Health Management and Economics at the Wharton School of the University of Pennsylvania. He has analyzed physician-organization integration for the past twenty-five years. In recognition of this research, he was named the Edwin L. Crosby Memorial Fellow by the Hospital Research and Educational Trust in 1992. He teaches courses on health care strategy, strategic change, and integrated delivery systems.

Lawrence P. Casalino, MD, PhD, is chief of the Division of Outcomes and Effectiveness Research at the Weill Cornell Medical College Department of Public Health. He worked for twenty years as a family physician in private practice, obtaining his PhD at University of California, Berkeley during the last few of those years. He is the recipient of an Investigator Award in Health Policy Research and has published more than fifty papers in leading medical journals.

Benjamin K. Chu, MD, MPH, MACP, is president of the Southern California Region of Kaiser Permanente. He currently directs health plan and hospital operations serving more than 3.2 million Kaiser Permanente members in southern California. Previously, he served as president of New York City's Health and Hospitals Corporation, the largest public hospital system in the country. He also currently serves on the board of The Commonwealth Fund and is chairman of the board of the American Legacy Foundation.

John R. Combes, MD, is a senior vice president of the American Hospital Association and president of the Center for Healthcare Governance, a trustee education and development company. He has more than 20 years of experience in executive health care leadership with deep expertise on issues relating to quality, patient safety, and medical ethics. He is a trustee for the Hospital Sisters Health System (a 13-hospital system) and chair of their quality committee.

James A. DeNuccio is director of Organized Medical Staff Services and Physicians in Practice, American Medical Association. Prior to joining the AMA, he served as vice president of operations for Advocate Christ Medical Center in Oak Lawn, Illinois, and senior vice president and chief operating officer of West Suburban Medical Center in Oak Park, Illinois, as well as other hospital senior-management positions.

Elliott S. Fisher, MD, MPH, is professor of Medicine and Community Family Medicine at Dartmouth Medical School. He received his undergraduate and medical degrees from Harvard University and was a Robert Wood Johnson Clinical Scholar at the University of Washington. He has served on the National Advisory Council of the Agency for Healthcare Research and Quality and now chairs a committee of the National Quality Forum.

Bruce J. Genovese, MD, MHSA, is co-chief medical information officer at Michigan Heart/Michigan Heart and Vascular Institute. He has been in a group cardiology practice for thirty-two years in Michigan and has held hospital administrative roles for twenty-five years. He has led the local physician organization and physician hospital organization. He has been a national business health care consultant for several years, focusing on physician-hospital alignment. He attended Georgetown University for his undergraduate degree and for medical school and the University of Michigan School of Public Health for his MHSA.

Jeff C. Goldsmith, PhD, is president of Health Futures, Inc. and associate professor of public health sciences at the University of Virginia. Previously, he was a lecturer at the University of Chicago on health services management and policy for eleven years. He has also lectured at the Harvard Business School, Wharton School, Johns Hopkins, and University of California, Berkeley. Additionally, he received the Dean Conley Award from the American College of Healthcare Executives for best health care article in 1985, 1990, and 1995.

Stuart Guterman, MA, is assistant vice president for The Commonwealth Fund's Program on Medicare's Future and is responsible for the research agenda related to the current performance and future improvements in the health payment system. He holds an AB in economics from Rutgers College and an MA in economics from Brown University.

Darrell G. Kirch, MD, is president and CEO of the Association of American Medical Colleges. A distinguished physician, educator, and medical scientist, he is also a noted authority on the organization and management of academic medical centers. His career spans all aspects of academic medicine and includes leadership positions at two medical schools and teaching hospitals and also at the National Institutes of Health.

Robert F. Leibenluft is a partner in Hogan & Hartson LLP. His practice is devoted entirely to antitrust matters in the health care sector. He headed the Health Care Division of the Federal Trade Commission's Bureau of Competition in the mid-1990s and is a former vice president of the American Health Lawyers Association and chair of the Health Care Committee of the American Bar Association Section of Antitrust Law. He currently serves on the board of directors of Prometheus Payment, Inc.

Ralph W. Muller, MA, is CEO of the University of Pennsylvania Health System (UPHS), Perelman Center for Advanced Medicine. Prior to joining UPHS, he was president and CEO of the University of Chicago Hospitals and Health System and a visiting fellow at the Kings Fund in London. He has served and currently serves on the boards of several national health care organizations.

David Posch, MS, is CEO for the Vanderbilt Clinic and executive director for the Vanderbilt Medical Group. Formerly, he worked at Ochsner Clinic in New Orleans for eight years, capping his career there as executive administrator. His career began at the Cleveland Clinic Foundation with sixteen years of progressive responsibilities in operations and strategic planning. He is a past member of the board of directors for the American Medical Group Association.

William M. Sage, MD, JD, is provost for health affairs and James R. Dougherty Chair for Faculty Excellence in Law at the University of Texas at Austin. He is an expert on health law and policy. Before assuming his current post, he was professor of law at Columbia University. He has written more than one hundred articles for legal, health policy, and clinical publications. He serves on the fellows council of the Hastings Center, a bioethics research institute, and is a member of the editorial board of *Health Affairs*.

Katherine A. Schneider, MD, MPhil, is vice president of health engagement at AtlantiCare. A family physician, she was previously chief medical officer of Integrated Resources of the Middlesex Area for Middlesex Health System, where she led participation in Medicare's Physician Group Practice Demonstration project. She has led several other projects around community health improvement and redesigning primary care, and she has received numerous awards for her leadership and teaching.

Anthony Shih, MD, MPH, is chief quality officer and vice president of strategic planning for IPRO, one of the nation's largest not-for-profit health care quality improvement organizations. He holds a BA in economics from Amherst College, an MD from the New York University School of Medicine, and an MPH from the Columbia University Mailman School of Public Health.

Stephen M. Shortell, PhD, MPH, is the Blue Cross of California Distinguished Professor of Health Policy and Management, professor of organization behavior, and dean at the School of Public Health at the University of California, Berkeley. A leading health care scholar, he has been the recipient of many awards, including the distinguished Baxter-Allegiance Prize, for his contributions to health services research.

Glenn D. Steele Jr., MD, PhD, is president and CEO of Geisinger Health System. He was previously the dean of the Biological Sciences division and the Pritzker School of Medicine and vice president for medical affairs at the University of Chicago. Prior to that, he was the William V. McDermott Professor of Surgery at Harvard Medical School, president and CEO of Deaconess Professional Practice Group, and chairman of the department of surgery at New England Deaconess Hospital (Boston). A prolific writer, he is the author or co-author of more than 460 scientific and professional articles.

Gary J. Young, PhD, JD, is professor and chair of the Department of Health Policy and Management at the Boston University School of Public Health. He is also associate director of the Boston University-affiliated Center for Organization, Leadership, and Management Research, which is funded by the Department of Veterans Affairs. His research focuses on management and legal issues associated with health care.

FOREWORD

Glenn D. Steele

As this book goes to press, it seems possible that the 2009/2010 health care reform debate will result in a significant expansion of access to health insurance. However, it is unlikely that health care delivery will be addressed directly by the present legislative process. Regardless of the outcome of the current debate, and even if no legislative changes occur in access or delivery, health care must and will be fundamentally redesigned in the near future for two reasons. First, the cost trajectory is unsustainable, given piece-rate payment incentives and a fragmented provider market that incorporates almost no widespread application of best practice or evidence-based care.[1] Second, the ethics of continuing to provide care that ensures no benefit and may actually harm 40 to 45 percent of patients is simply embarrassing, no matter how much profit a particular stakeholder can justify.[2]

For both economic and ethical reasons, the pressure to change care delivery will dramatically increase if, as a society, we do decide to cover a significant percentage of currently uninsured citizens with a minimally acceptable benefit package. Demand for health care services is likely to increase beyond what is now modeled in the various congressional proposals, just as it did in the Massachusetts reform experiment. If we continue to pay for units of work rather than outcomes (particularly if units are priced by political, not market-driven, processes), and if we meet most of the increased demand with the least efficient or effective provider sites (hospital emergency rooms), we can assume that the expense trajectory now being modeled is also vastly underestimated, just as it was in Massachusetts.

Quite apart from the cost issue, the ethical imperative to change how we provide care is now more widely accepted. The natural consequence of the Institute of Medicine's seminal focus on hospital mortality ten years ago and the subsequent local, regional, and national efforts to improve quality have shown that when goals are set and metrics are available and transparent, change will occur to the benefit of those we serve.[3]

So, if the time for fundamental care redesign is now, what should be changed? I would suggest the following targets: 1) unjustified variation in how we care for patients within a given institution or system and throughout the country as a whole; 2) fragmentation of care; 3) reimbursement for units of work, not for minimally acceptable outcomes; and 4) patients as passive recipients of care.[4]

Is there proof that any particular provider structure enables us to tackle these challenges or brings us closer to optimal, value based, patient-centric care? Perhaps. Certainly those of us who are immersed in truly integrated delivery systems believe that our quality and value outcomes are better for individual patients and perhaps for populations as well. A few academic investigators have begun to confirm this.[5] But there are other organizational structures that have evolved into superbly productive generators of medical education and basic medical knowledge. Their design is perfectly suited for an equally complex set of missions as the recently celebrated integrated delivery system models. Further, with some notable exceptions, few integrated delivery systems combine financial risk-taking or risk-spreading (in other words, the insurance function) with the delivery of a continuum of primary through hospital-based subspecialty care. This is also an important model; without such truly integrated health system functions (care delivery and financing), care redesign that benefits the patient often harms the patient's provider financially.

Even if we could come to a consensus about a perfect provider system structure or a limited number of optimal structures, how do we get from where we are to where we want to be without creating havoc? Many of the authors in this book represent health care institutions (either academic or integrated systems) that are organized very differently from the small physician practices and low-capacity hospitals that comprise the bulk of our U.S. health care universe. Is there a way of defining a limited number of optimal structures to provide better health outcomes at lower cost, learning from admittedly unusual models, and, in a trial and error process, attempting to scale and generalize to the more heterogeneous dominant marketplace?

No one template can possibly deliver a single optimal solution. However, for the common patient care mission shared by all providers, there must be an important shared predicate: to achieve fundamental redesign of care, providers will not only have to work together but in fact, serve as leaders of system change. Primary care physicians at the front door of any integrated system will need to work seamlessly with hospital-based specialists to provide quality and value over time to patients with acute or chronic care needs. Physicians and hospitals will need to work together within a single operational construct. And perhaps even insurance companies will need to work with providers (both physicians and hospitals), not simply to negotiate acceptable "piece rate" reimbursement, but to reframe the conversation as to how best to achieve optimal outcomes for specific subpopulations of their patients/members.

I am certain that the concept of professional "pride of purpose" remains a latent but powerful motivation to rethink how we care for patients. What most often neutralizes this core value is the frantic day-to-day struggle to survive, either financially or academically. I would imagine that, as a primary care physician, it is difficult to think creatively about ways to better care for patients if you are simply struggling to expand your panel or maximize the frequency of high financial yield ancillary services to send your children to college. Likewise, if you are running a relatively small hospital with no access to capital and marginally successful operations, innovation is not at the top of your "to do" list. The question then becomes how does a better structural context allow for realization of this "pride of purpose" for a greater portion of our provider community?

This book begins to elucidate where we have been, where we are now, and a bit of where we should go to create structures that might unleash provider-driven, patient-focused, value-based care redesign. If we truly aspire (or are forced) to become a system capable of delivering health services that optimize individual patient and population outcomes, our structures will need to resemble those of a number of integrated delivery systems or integrated health systems, or at the very least we will need to create a virtual approximation in the near term. What follows is an excellent start in claiming an intellectual premise for that journey.

Notes

1. The Commonwealth Fund Commission on a High Performance Health System, *The Path to a High Performance U.S. Health System: A 2020 Vision and the Policies to Pave the Way* (New York: The Commonwealth Fund, 2009), 16–21.
2. E. A. McGlenn, S. M. Asch, J. Adams, J. Jeesey, and others, "The Quality of Health Care Delivered to Adults in the United States," *New England Journal of Medicine* 348, no. 26 (June 26, 2003): 2635–45.
3. Institute of Medicine, *To Err Is Human: Building a Safer Health System* (Washington, D.C.: National Academies Press, 2000); A. S. Casale, R. A. Paulus, M. J. Selna, and others.

"ProvenCare®: A Provider-Driven Pay-for-Performance Program for Acute Episodic Cardiac Surgical Care," *Annals of Surgery* 246, no. 4 (2007): 270–80; D. McCarthy, S.K.H. How, C. Schoen, J. C. Cantor, and others, *Aiming Higher: Results from a State Scorecard on Health System Performance, 2009* (New York: The Commonwealth Fund, October 2009), http://www.commonwealthfund.org/~/media/Files/Publications/Fund%20Report/2009/Oct/1326_McCarthy_state_scorecard_2009_full_report_FINAL.pdf.

4. R. A. Paulus, K. Davis, and G. D. Steele, "Continuous Innovation in Health Care: Implications of the Geisinger Experience," *Health Affairs* 27, no. 5 (September–October 2008): 1235–45.

5. D. R. Rittenhouse, L. P. Casalino, R. R. Gillies, S. M. Shortell, and others, "Measuring the Medical Home Infrastructure in Large Medical Groups," *Health Affairs* 27, no. 5 (September–October 2008): 1246–58.

PARTNERS IN HEALTH

CHAPTER ONE

INTRODUCTION AND VISION

Francis J. Crosson
Laura A. Tollen

Introduction

As this book goes to press, the United States is in the midst of a multiyear struggle to design and implement comprehensive health care reform. As a nation, we have embarked on a journey of sensibility and equity that has been too long delayed. The end of this journey is obscure, but before it is over and a new equilibrium established, the journey will engage nearly every person and institution in the country. This book is an attempt to describe one important element of that eventual equilibrium—the physician-hospital relationship—and by doing so the authors hope to speed along the journey itself.

It has been estimated that expansion of health care coverage to 90 percent or more of U.S. citizens will cost in excess of one trillion dollars in the first ten years. This figure may prove to be a significant underestimate. Higher than expected costs from the Massachusetts near-universal coverage experiment have contributed to a potential four billion dollar budget shortfall in that state for 2010. For U.S health care reform to be politically successful, individually affordable, and nationally sustainable, it must contain the elements necessary to constrain cost growth. This will require a reduction of the annual average health care cost increase from more than 2 percent above the annual growth in gross domestic product (GDP) to between zero and 1 percent above GDP growth. The alternative is a significant increase in federal revenues through taxation. Although this task might not seem daunting when expressed in terms of a 1 or 2 percent change in the rate of expenditure growth, such a change will involve billions of dollars of cost reductions annually and have a major impact on all parts of the health care industry.

Any approach to sustained cost reduction in health care must involve hospitals and physicians. Hospitalizations are the most costly form of care delivery, and conventional wisdom is that physician care decisions directly drive over 80 percent of total health care costs. Accordingly, there is a growing consensus that changes in payment incentives to hospitals and physicians are required, and that such changes must be more than superficial.[1] Most such payment reforms involve either prepayment for services to be rendered, with some form of risk sharing, or episode-based payments such as case payments to physicians and hospitals together.

But there is a problem. As seen in Figure 1.1, advanced payment methodologies are most feasible in an environment of highly organized providers.[2] Such payment methodologies are much less feasible in the disaggregated delivery model that exists in much of the United States today. Most small physician offices are not capable of managing prepayment risk, nor should they be. Capitation of small

FIGURE 1.1 ORGANIZATION AND PAYMENT METHODS

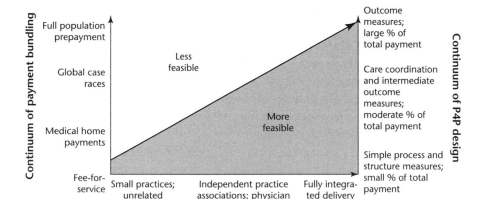

Source: A. Shih, K. Davis, S. Schoenbaum, A. Gauthier, R. Nuzum, and D. McCarthy, "Organizing the U.S. Health Care Delivery System for High Performance" (New York: The Commonwealth Fund, August 2008), Exhibit ES-1, p. xi, http://www.commonwealthfund.org/Content/Publications/Fund-Reports/2008/Aug/Organizing-the-U-S--Health-Care-Delivery-System-for-High-Performance.aspx. Reproduced with permission of The Commonwealth Fund.

physician groups was shown to be unstable in the 1990s and presented significant ethical concerns. Similarly, few U.S. hospitals have sufficient integration with their physician staffs to be able to accept episode-based payments without considerable rancor and physician opposition, and potential violations of several federal regulations (see Chapter Six).

The solution to the problem is a coordinated set of delivery system reforms that involve changes in both payment and incentives and in the structure of how hospitals and physicians are organized to provide care. The changes must address the chicken-or-the-egg dilemma that has impeded progress in delivery system integration in many parts of the country. Without payment reform, there is little motivation for disaggregated physicians to do the hard work of forming larger organizations and to work with hospital administrators. Conversely, without the existence of greater numbers of integrated organizations, payers (including Medicare) have gained little traction in developing advanced payment methodologies because so few entities are capable of receiving them and succeeding with them.

Over the past eighty years, there have been a number of carefully constructed calls for delivery system integration (or *organization*, as shown in Figure 1.1). In 1933, the Committee on the Costs of Medical Care recommended that the United States seek to create many more group practices (modeled after the Mayo Clinic), because such practices were more efficient and less costly than solo practices.[3] More recently, the Institute of Medicine, in its report *Crossing the Quality Chasm: A New Health System for the 21st Century*, identified six "redesign imperatives" for future care delivery in the United States: redesigned care processes; effective use of information technologies; knowledge and skills management; development of effective teams; coordination of care across patient conditions, services, and settings over time; and use of performance and outcome measurement for continuous quality improvement and accountability.[4] The strong implication of the report was that significant structural change was needed in care delivery to achieve these process characteristics.

Finally, in its landmark report in 2007, *A High Performance Health System for the United States*, The Commonwealth Fund Commission on a High Performance Health System called for "the U.S. [to] embark on the organization and delivery of health care services to end the fragmentation, waste, and complexity that currently exist. Physicians and other care providers should be rewarded, through financial and non-financial incentives, to band together into traditional or virtual organizations that can provide the support needed for physicians and other providers to practice 21st century medicine."[5]

The goal then, in the context of Figure 1.1, is to move through both payment changes and delivery system changes over time from the "southwest" corner of the figure to somewhere closer to the "northeast" corner. There are many ideas about how to do this, discussed throughout this book. Virtually every one of these ideas for change will require increased collaboration or integration between hospitals and physicians. The purpose of this book is to describe what will need to change in the relationships between these providers to drive movement from disaggregation through collaboration to integration.

Delivery System Reform Proposals

In 2009, anticipating some type of national health reform, various stakeholders developed delivery system reform proposals to achieve the goals referred to earlier. Most of these require changes in the relationships between hospitals and physicians to be effective. Here, we will discuss three of these proposals:

- Clinical integration, as envisioned by the American Hospital Association (AHA)[6]
- Bundled payments to physicians and hospitals, as recommended by the Medicare Payment Advisory Commission (MedPAC)[7]
- Accountable care organizations (ACOs), as conceptualized by MedPAC, the Brookings Institution, and others[8]

Clinical Integration

Most U.S. physicians practice medicine, at least in part, within a hospital setting but without a direct legal or financial relationship with the hospital. There are some exceptions to this model. In integrated delivery systems, such as Kaiser Permanente, the Mayo Clinic, and the Geisinger Health System, most physicians are employed by the group practice, which either owns or has a financial arrangement with the hospital or hospitals. Similarly, in physician hospital organizations (PHOs), the hospital and its associated physicians create a joint financial entity through which revenue is distributed. Recently, hospitals have begun to employ physicians directly in a variety of specialties. Some of this change has come about because of hospitals' difficulty in finding physicians willing to cover emergency services after hours and because of the rapid growth of hospitalist programs.[9]

In each of these settings, there is usually a sound structural, financial, and legal basis for physicians to work closely together to improve care quality and reduce unnecessary costs. For example, in Kaiser Permanente, orthopedic surgeons regularly analyze the success rates of various artificial hip devices, determine which ones are best for patient care, and agree to use only those devices. In turn, this agreement allows the hospital to achieve economies of scale on the purchase of these devices.

In the more common setting, where the physicians and hospitals are not part of a single economic entity, the situation is quite different. In some states, the "corporate practice of medicine bar" prevents hospitals from hiring physicians (except in certain specialties such as pathology), even if the physicians wish to be employed. In addition, a broad range of federal laws and regulations inhibits physician-hospital interrelationships, including antitrust provisions, tax-exempt organization regulations, laws intended to prevent limitation of services to Medicare beneficiaries, and "anti-kickback" and "Stark" provisions.[10] These regulations, as well as possible mitigation approaches, are discussed in detail in Chapter Six.

To improve physician-hospital collaboration in settings where physicians and hospitals are not part of an economic entity, the AHA Task Force on Delivery System Fragmentation recommended that the AHA seek ways to integrate clinical care across providers, across settings, and over time.[11] The task force called for the federal government to "establish a simpler, consistent set of rules for how hospitals and physicians conduct their working relationships. The complexity, inconsistency and sometimes conflicting interpretations of federal laws and regulations affecting physician-hospital arrangements are a significant barrier. Few arrangements can be structured without significant legal expense."[12]

Subsequent AHA-sponsored work has identified a number of goals for clinical integration:

- Foster collaboration to improve quality of care.
- Improve quality and efficiency for independent providers.
- Enable providers to perform well in pay-for-performance and other public reporting initiatives.
- Gain experience in forming provider organizations responsible for an entire episode of care or population of patients.
- Provide a vehicle for a hospital to work more closely with members of its medical staff.
- Provide the means whereby providers can obtain greater reimbursement to cover the added costs of their efforts and that recognize the increased value of the services they offer.[13]

In response to the AHA efforts, the Federal Trade Commission (FTC) held a workshop with the AHA to examine the topic of clinical integration and the potential for changes in federal laws and regulation that could remove perceived barriers to such integration efforts. However, in late April 2009, FTC

Commissioner Pamela Jones Harbour told the AHA that the FTC would not be issuing clarifying rules, or "safe harbors," regarding clinical integration but would continue to issue case-by-case judgments.[14]

On the other hand, MedPAC has recommended to Congress that it enact changes to existing laws and regulations to allow *gainsharing* between hospitals and physicians for specified activities intended to improve quality and increase efficiency.[15] As part of the Deficit Reduction Act of 2005, Congress authorized and the Centers for Medicare and Medicaid Services (CMS) subsequently implemented two gainsharing demonstration projects, which are still pending completion and evaluation.

Were there to be a significant "relaxation" of the laws and regulations that now inhibit financial arrangements between otherwise separate physicians and hospitals, it is possible that more formal integrated structures such as those that we will discuss later in this chapter might be less necessary. However, the pace of such regulatory changes is likely to be too slow to foster the type of systematic reorganization that appears to be called for now, as part of health care reform. Therefore, other, more complex proposals are under consideration.

Bundled Payments

Currently, physicians and hospitals that are financially independent of each other are paid separately. For example, Medicare pays most acute care hospitals through the Medicare Part A Prospective Payment System (PPS), based upon case rates known as diagnosis-related groups (DRGs). Physicians are paid for services provided in both the hospital and office settings through the Medicare Part B resource-based relative value scale (see Chapter Four).

The incentives inherent in these two payment systems are not aligned. Once a Medicare beneficiary is admitted for care, the hospital, which is to receive a fixed payment for that hospitalization, has an incentive to deliver services efficiently and to avoid unnecessarily prolonging the hospitalization. The physicians caring for the beneficiary, on the other hand, will be paid by Medicare for each service they deliver, irrespective of the complexity of the service or the length of the hospitalization. Thus, there is no financial incentive for the physicians to be efficient, and as noted earlier, generally the hospital is prevented by law from providing such incentives. In addition, there is no financial incentive for physicians to work together during the hospitalization to avoid duplication of services.

To address this problem, some payers have tried to combine payments to physicians and hospitals in a model known as *bundling*, or episode-based payments. Payments can be bundled for multiple services delivered by one provider, such as a payment that covers admissions and readmissions for the same condition.

Payments can also be bundled for services provided by multiple providers, such as physicians and hospitals. It is this latter form of bundling that we address here. In the early 1990s, Medicare created the Medicare Participating Heart Bypass Center Demonstration, which bundled hospital and physician payments for cardiac bypass graft surgery (see Chapters Four and Five). The payments covered readmissions within seventy-two hours postdischarge and related physician services for a ninety-day period. Although the demonstration was considered successful, it was not renewed because of opposition from some parts of the hospital industry. However, more recently, the Geisinger Health System in Pennsylvania instituted a similar bundled payment initiative called ProvenCare, which resulted in a 44 percent drop in readmissions over the first eighteen months.[16]

In its June 2008 report, MedPAC, having studied the issue for more than a year, made three unanimous recommendations to Congress regarding bundling. These recommendations were as follows:

- **Recommendation 4A**—The Congress should require the [U.S.] Secretary [of Health and Human Services] to confidentially report readmission rates to hospitals and physicians. Beginning in the third year, providers' relative resource use should be publicly disclosed.
- **Recommendation 4B**—To encourage providers to collaborate and better coordinate care, the Congress should direct the Secretary to reduce payments to hospitals with relatively high readmission rates for select conditions and also allow shared accountability between physicians and hospitals. The Congress should also direct the Secretary to report within two years on the feasibility of broader approaches, such as virtual bundling, for encouraging efficiency around hospitalization episodes.
- **Recommendation 4C**—The Congress should require the Secretary to create a voluntary pilot program to test the feasibility of actual bundled payment for services around hospitalization episodes for select conditions. The pilot must have clear and explicit thresholds for determining whether it can be expanded into the full Medicare program or should be discontinued.[17]

The MedPAC commissioners had three behavior changes in mind in making this set of recommendations. First, the commissioners believed, based on research regarding geographic variation in the frequency of physician inpatient visits during hospitalization, that bundling could provide the incentive and opportunity for physicians to reduce the number of hospital visits without harming quality.[18] Second, they intended that a bundled payment pilot would remove legal barriers that currently keep hospitals from compensating physicians for using fewer resources during a hospital stay. Third, depending upon the structure of the bundled payment, physicians would be encouraged to focus on posthospital care and the prevention of readmissions. (The MedPAC commissioners found that up to 80 percent of Medicare readmissions might be preventable with better coordination of acute care and postacute care services.)

MedPAC envisioned that bundled payments could be "virtual"; in other words, physicians and hospitals would receive separate payments that would be equally adjusted up or down based on their collective performance relative to national or local benchmarks. Actual bundled payments would be tested on a voluntary basis through a pilot program, in part because these payments require the creation of an agreement between physicians and hospitals regarding how the payment is to be divided. Such arrangements would be difficult to mandate. On the other hand, actual bundling is a stronger model precisely because it forces a close working relationship between the hospital and the medical staff.

Whichever model proves to be the best, this type of incentive change is difficult. As noted by Glenn Hackbarth, MedPAC's chairman, "MedPAC is under no illusion that the path of policy change outlined here is easy. Unforeseen consequences are likely, and midcourse adjustments will be needed. But a continuation of the status quo is unacceptable. The current payment system is fueling many of the worst aspects of our health care system, leaving beneficiaries' care uncoordinated, and increasing health care costs to an extent that strains many beneficiaries' ability to pay their health bills, the nation's ability to finance Medicare, and the ability of a large segment of the non-Medicare population to afford health insurance."[19]

Following the recommendation by MedPAC, the Secretary of the Department of Health and Human Services authorized the creation of the Medicare Acute Care Episode Demonstration, which began in 2009. Five hospitals in the states of New Mexico, Oklahoma, Texas, and Colorado volunteered to receive bundled payments for specified cardiovascular and orthopedic services. Gainsharing between the hospitals and the medical staff is allowed, and there are beneficiary incentives in the form of reduced out-of-pocket expenses. Further, at the end of 2009 it appeared possible that Congress would require bundling of payments to participating Medicare hospitals in 2014 as part of larger health reform efforts.

Accountable Care Organizations

In 2003 the physician leaders of thirty-four of the nation's largest multispecialty group practices formed the Council of Accountable Physician Practices (CAPP) to focus attention on what they believed was the most successful delivery system model in the United States.[20] These groups included, for example, the Permanente

Medical Groups, the Mayo Clinic, the Geisinger Health System, the Henry Ford Health System, and Intermountain Health Care. Most of these group practices either owned hospitals or had close working relationships with one or more hospitals. In addition, they were strong believers in the improved performance possible with physician-hospital integration. Over the next five years, CAPP sponsored research into the relative performance in quality and efficiency of such groups compared to disaggregated practices.[21] In 2008 Tollen reviewed the literature on the subject and found that, in general, there was a positive correlation between practice organization and better performance.[22]

In light of the experience of the CAPP medical groups and the developing data that supported claims of better results, in 2005 Crosson called for the inclusion of structural reform of the delivery system, similar to such integrated delivery systems, in any future attempt at comprehensive health care reform.[23] The obvious problem was that there were not enough such delivery systems in existence to cover more than a fifth of the U.S. population, and most were concentrated in the West and Midwest regions of the country.

In 2006 Fisher and colleagues proposed a solution to this problem.[24] Noticing that most Medicare beneficiaries received most of their care from a single primary care provider and the hospital(s) in which that provider most often practiced, the authors proposed that integrated delivery systems could be created quickly by having payers "assign" patients to hospitals and their "extended medical staffs" based upon such usage patterns. They called the resulting virtually integrated system an accountable care organization (ACO). In 2008 Shortell and Casalino sought to broaden the model under the term *accountable care systems* (ACSs) and called for payment reforms to create incentives for more such organizations.[25] In 2009 Fisher and colleagues refined the ACO model and laid out a five-year reform schedule for Medicare to institute payment to ACOs.[26] Note that this book will use the term *accountable care organization* in a general sense to refer to the broad concept of an entity that is clinically and fiscally accountable for the entire continuum of care that patients may need, rather than to any specific ACO model that has been proposed. (Any exceptions to this usage have been noted by the authors of individual chapters.)

In its June 2009 report to Congress, MedPAC reported on more than a year of study and analysis of the ACO concept, laying the groundwork for potential legislation that would move the Medicare program in this direction.[27] As the report states, "By giving physicians and hospitals a way to increase their income through ACO-wide quality improvement and reducing unnecessary services, the Medicare system would gain a way to constrain spending other than through the blunt instrument of lowering FFS [fee-for-service] updates. . . . For Medicare to become sustainable, the delivery system has to change.

ACOs could prove to be an important catalyst for delivery system reform by creating incentives for increased organization and joint decision making."[28]

At the end of 2009 Congress seemed intent on creating robust pilot testing of ACOs and accompanying payment changes as part of a reformed Medicare program. However Congress and the Secretary choose to support and implement ACOs in the future, physician-hospital integration will be required to make the model work. The more comprehensive the reform and the faster the change in payment incentives evolves, the more important will be the development of the knowledge base for making this change successful. As noted by Crosson, "a successful movement to the availability of ACOs will require substantial changes in how physicians and hospitals relate to and seek to integrate with each other. Integration must occur at the operational, financial, and cultural levels, each of which faces a number of barriers."[29]

Physician-Hospital Integration as Central to Delivery System Reform

Whether the AHA model of clinical integration, integration driven by a more widespread use of bundled payments, or the evolution of ACOs becomes the predominant reform dynamic in the next five or so years, there is little question that change is coming. The well-known *Dartmouth Atlas* data have made it abundantly clear that health care services are unnecessarily expensive and of poor quality in many parts of the country.[30] There are really only two ways to reduce those costs, either through progressive fee-for-service payment reductions to physicians and hospitals or through reorganization of care delivery and changes to payment and incentives. It is likely that only the latter choice has a simultaneous chance to improve quality.

So the best hope is the most radical—to restructure and integrate. But are U.S. physicians and hospitals capable of proceeding successfully through such changes? The old medical staff model seems to be failing, for reasons discussed later in this book. Some institutions, such as the multispecialty group practices mentioned earlier, are ready and waiting to thrive on new payment models. But most hospitals and their medical staffs are not. Some remember all too well the failed attempts to "integrate" in the mid-1990s to prepare for managed care prepayment, which never materialized. Many nascent organizations failed or disbanded as a consequence. Hard feelings and financial losses were the result. Currently, in many institutions, physicians and hospitals are at loggerheads over control issues or are in frank competition for patients needing complex, profitable procedures.

A first step in breaking down this negative environment is to analyze what is wrong and how it could be different. There are many aspects to solving this problem—clinical, legal, financial, psychological, and cultural, to name a few. These various aspects of the problem and solutions to them have not been brought together in one place before. That is the goal of this book.

About This Book

Some of the needed experience and knowledge to bridge the physician-hospital divide exists in the health care academic community, among individuals who have devoted their lives to gaining understanding, teaching, and creating new knowledge. Some of the needed experience and knowledge exists in the practical fact base of delivery system leaders, who have devoted their lives to building and improving real-world institutions of care delivery. This book is designed to be read by, and to be of value to, members of both these constituencies. Accordingly, the authors have been selected from among the most distinguished individuals in both of these disciplines. The book is intended to contain both academic analyses and real-world examples of successful change. The book can be read as individual chapters, but it is intended, ideally, to be read as an entirety—to tell a story of change that is multifaceted and difficult but also necessary and possible.

In Chapter Two, "History of Physician-Hospital Collaboration: Obstacles and Opportunities," Lawton Burns, of the Wharton School of Business, Jeff Goldsmith of Health Futures, and Ralph Muller of the University of Pennsylvania Health System review the changes in physician-hospital relationships during the twentieth century. Based on their analysis of this history, they argue that the major provider-based competencies called for in health care reform may best be satisfied by hospitals rather than physicians. They also note that hospitals' past attempts to collaborate more closely with physicians have relied heavily on structural mechanisms, such as salaried employment, leadership roles, and contracting vehicles. However, there is little evidence that the use of these mechanisms has helped the pursuit of value. As a result, hospitals and the physicians with which they work will need to carefully consider the factors that have prevented more significant behavioral change. These factors, each explored throughout this book, include real and perceived legal barriers, differences in culture between hospitals and physicians (and among physicians), and major differences in governance structures.

In Chapter Three, "Achieving the Vision: Structural Change," Stephen Shortell of the University of California, Berkeley, Lawrence Casalino of Cornell, and Elliott Fisher of Dartmouth describe the range of proposed structural or organizational models for promoting greater alignment and integration between hospitals and physicians. They call these models, collectively, "accountable care organizations." They begin with an overview of the aspects of institutional culture that differentiate hospitals from physician organizations, describing the inherent conflict between bureaucracy and professional autonomy. Next, they analyze four models of accountable care systems: the integrated delivery system, the multispecialty group practice, the physician hospital organization, and the independent practice association. Each of these models has varying potential for promoting greater collaboration between hospitals and physicians. The key is the extent to which they can take advantage of possible new payment incentives to develop commitment to shared goals and the capabilities to realize those goals. In conclusion, the authors discuss the need for supportive financial incentives and changes in the regulatory or legal environment to foster the development and success of accountable care organizations.

In Chapter Four, "Achieving the Vision: Payment Reform," Stuart Guterman of The Commonwealth Fund and Anthony Shih of IPRO analyze a range of payment reform proposals designed to encourage the type of structural integration between hospitals and physicians described in the previous chapter. Their chapter describes how the evolution of payment methods and other market factors have affected the "traditional" hospital medical staff model. This is followed by a discussion of payment methodologies that are viewed as potentially useful in appropriately aligning hospital and physician incentives with the patient's best interest. These include hospital pay-for-performance, shared savings, blended payment for primary care, and episode-based payments. Ultimately, the authors suggest that payers should adopt a flexible payment approach—one that offers an array of alternative payment models that incentivize quality and efficiency through various levels of bundling matched to the capabilities of the current organizational structures.

In Chapter Five, "Achieving the Vision: Operational Challenges and Improvement," Bruce Genovese of the Michigan Heart and Vascular Institute outlines the operational value and clinical capabilities of highly functioning integrated organizations, as well as the obstacles to such capabilities that exist in many delivery sites across the country today. He describes potential solutions for such obstacles, including common clinical information technology platforms and common performance measurements and goals. Genovese also provides a case study of a successful physician-hospital collaboration in Michigan (Saint Joseph Mercy Hospital's participation in the Medicare Participating Heart Bypass Center Demonstration), focusing on the operational enablers and benefits.

The change to ACOs, which will be built on physician-hospital integration, is likely to be a ten- to fifteen-year proposition. It will face a series of barriers, any one of which could derail such change. We know this from observation of the failures, as well as the occasional successes of the physician hospital organization (PHO) movement in the 1990s. In the next three chapters, the authors describe these barriers and potential solutions to or pathways around them.

In Chapter Six, "Overcoming Barriers to Improved Collaboration and Alignment: Legal and Regulatory Issues," Robert Leibenluft of Hogan and Hartson and William Sage of the University of Texas, Austin, focus on the extent to which legal change is necessary for significant health care reform. The chapter begins with an examination of federal antitrust laws and their perceived and real impact on physician-hospital collaboration. The authors discuss potential barriers to the formation of ACOs and also some of the antitrust issues that might arise if a particular ACO became dominant in a given geographic area. Next, the authors examine two other important federal issues: fraud and abuse, and tax exemption. They discuss several state laws that affect hospitals' and physicians' ability to improve collaboration, including health professional licensing and scope of practice, the corporate practice of medicine doctrine and physician employment, medical staff credentialing, insurance regulation, and medical malpractice. The authors conclude with a series of key questions regarding the legal environment that should guide the health care reform debate.

In Chapter Seven, "Overcoming Barriers to Improved Collaboration and Alignment: Governance Issues," Jeffrey Alexander of the University of Michigan and Gary Young of Boston University review the historical development of hospital governing boards and medical staffs, and discuss how regulation, reimbursement, and competition have shaped relations between the two groups. The chapter next considers internal and external factors that have impeded alignment between hospital governing boards and medical staffs. Next, the authors analyze several strategies to enable hospital and medical staff governing entities to take a leading role in promoting alignment between hospitals and physicians. These include development of "workaround" organizations such as physician hospital organizations (PHOs), foundations, and joint ventures. The chapter concludes with several policy recommendations. In addition, James DeNuccio of the American Medical Association and John R. Combes of the American Hospital Association provide brief perspective commentaries.

In Chapter Eight, "Overcoming Barriers to Improved Collaboration and Alignment: Cultural Issues," Katherine Schneider of AtlantiCare uses her experience in creating the physician hospital organization at Middlesex Hospital in Connecticut (the only non-group-practice entity to qualify as a Medicare Group Practice Demonstration site) to explore the range of human dynamics that have prevented closer collaboration and innovation between hospitals and practicing physicians. She also describes what she calls "rules for engagement" for hospitals hoping to entice physicians to enter into new collaborative ventures, asserting that physicians will not allow their time and attention to be diverted from patient care unless the proposed collaboration will do at least one of the following: save them time, add value to their patients' experience, increase their income or improve their quality of life, or add to their professional satisfaction. Conversely, there are rules for engagement on the hospital side as well. Schneider notes that in order for engagement with physicians to be worth administrators' efforts, the activity must be consistent with the organization's mission, vision, values, and strategy; result in improvement in a key measurable outcome, without adversely affecting another measure; and result in increased happiness of one key stakeholder without resulting in ire from another one. Further, the operational requirements and implications of the activity must be adequately identified, and it must be possible to accommodate them. Schneider concludes with a series of recommendations for bridging the cultural divide between hospitals and physicians to encourage collaboration for quality and efficiency.

Not all hospitals in the United States are the same. Among other differences are variations in geography, financial base, and mission that separate institutions. Such differences can create particular strengths and weaknesses relative to physician-hospital integration. The authors of the next two chapters explore the special issues of safety net providers and explore special issues for safety net providers and academic medical centers in the context of the goals outlined in this book.

In Chapter Nine, "Special Issues for Safety Net Hospitals and Clinics," Benjamin Chu of Kaiser Permanente, formerly of the New York City Health and Hospitals Corporation, examines the special issues of public health care providers, especially those in large city environments. He focuses on two real examples of physician-hospital integration in safety net institutions, Denver Health and the New York City organization that he led and improved. Chu generalizes from these examples to a set of principles that can help guide other such institutions, as well as non-safety-net providers that are seeking to change in a similar fashion.

In Chapter Ten, "Special Issues for Academic Medical Centers," David Posch of Vanderbilt University Medical Center addresses, in similar fashion, the range of considerations facing academic medical centers that seek to create "group practices" out of disparate clinician/teacher/researcher physicians at such institutions. Drawing on his experience at Vanderbilt, he provides recommendations for the future of academic hospitals. Darrell Kirch of the Association of American Medical Colleges provides a commentary on this chapter.

Finally, in Chapter Eleven, "What Needs to Happen Next?" Francis Crosson draws from and highlights the knowledge brought forth in the preceding chapters. In collaboration with the other chapter authors and the information gleaned from a set of workshops that accompanied the creation of this book, he describes a cascade of potential legislative, regulatory, voluntary operational, and market-driven changes that could, in combination, bring about the development and success of new models of physician-hospital integration, as part of a reformed, twenty-first century health care system.

Notes

1. P. B. Ginsburg, "Provider Payment Incentives and Delivery System Reform," in *The Health Care Delivery System: A Blueprint for Reform* (Washington, D.C.: Center for American Progress and the Institute on Medicine as a Profession, 2008); A. Shih, K. Davis, S. C. Schoenbaum, A. Gauthier, and others, *Organizing the U.S. Health Care Delivery System for High Performance* (New York: The Commonwealth Fund, 2008), http://www.commonwealthfund .org/Content/Publications/Fund-Reports/2008/Aug/Organizing-the-U-S--Health-Care-Delivery-System-for-High-Performance.aspx.

2. Shih and others, *Organizing the U.S. Health Care Delivery System for High Performance*, Exhibit ES-1, p. xi.

3. I. S. Falk, C. R. Rorem, and M. D Ring, *The Costs of Medical Care: A Summary of Investigations on the Economic Aspects of the Prevention and Care of Illness* (Chicago: University of Chicago Press, 1933).

4. Institute of Medicine, *Crossing the Quality Chasm: A New Health System for the 21st Century* (Washington, D.C.: National Academies Press, 2001), 119–54.

5. Commonwealth Fund Commission on a High Performance Health System, *A High Performance Health System for the United States: An Ambitious Agenda for the Next President* (New York: The Commonwealth Fund, 2007), p. 28, http://www.commonwealthfund.org/ Content/Publications/Fund-Reports/2007/Nov/A-High-Performance-Health-System-for-the-United-States--An-Ambitious-Agenda-for-the-Next-President.aspx.

6. American Hospital Association (AHA), *Aligning Hospital and Physician Interests: Broadening the Concept of Gain Sharing to Allow Care Improvement Incentives* (Chicago: American Hospital Association, 2005), attachment A/2.

7. Medicare Payment Advisory Commission (MedPAC), "A Path to Bundled Payment Around a Hospitalization," in *Report to the Congress: Reforming the Delivery System* (Washington, D.C.: Medicare Payment Advisory Commission, 2008), 83–106.

8. MedPAC, "Accountable Care Organizations," in *Report to the Congress: Improving Incentives in the Medicare Program* (Washington, D.C.: Medicare Payment Advisory Commission, 2009) 39–60, http://www.medpac.gov/chapters/June09_Ch01.pdf; E. S. Fisher M. B. McClellan, J. Bertko, S. M. Lieberman, and others, "Fostering Accountable Health Care: Moving Forward in Medicare," *Health Affairs* Web exclusive (January 27, 2009), w219–w231, http:// content.healthaffairs.org/cgi/reprint/hlthaff.28.2.w219v1.

9. R. A. Berenson, P. A. Ginsburg, and J. H. May, "Hospital-Physician Relations: Cooperation, Competition, or Separation?" *Health Affairs* Web exclusive (December 5, 2006), w31–w43, http://content.healthaffairs.org/cgi/reprint/26/1/w31.

10. T. S. Jost and E. J. Emanuel, "Legal Reforms Necessary to Promote Delivery System Innovation," *JAMA* 299, no. 21 (2009): 2561–63.

11. American Hospital Association, "Modernizing Gain Sharing Opportunities: Recommendations of the Task Force on Delivery System Fragmentation" (2005), p. 2, http://www.aha.org/aha/content/2007/pdf/modernizinggainshare.pdf.

12. American Hospital Association, "Modernizing Gain Sharing Opportunities."

13. T. Leary, R. B. Leibenluft, S. Pozen, and T. E. Weir, "Guidance for Clinical Integration: Working Paper" (Hogan and Hartson, LLP, for the American Hospital Association, April 2007).

14. P. Harbour, Federal Trade Commissioner, "Clinical Integration: The Changing Policy Climate and What It Means for Care Coordination" (speech before the American Hospital Association, Washington, D.C., April 27, 2009).

15. MedPAC, *Report to the Congress: Reforming the Delivery System* (Statement by Mark E. Miller, Ph.D., executive director of the Medicare Payment Advisory Commission, to the Committee on Finance, U.S. Senate, September 16, 2008), p. 15, http://www.medpac.gov/documents/20080916_Sen%20Fin_testimony%20final.pdf.

16. R. E. Mechanic and S. H. Altman, "Payment Reform Options: Episode Payment Is the Place to Start," *Health Affairs* Web exclusive (Jan. 27, 2009), w262–w271. http://content.healthaffairs.org/cgi/reprint/28/2/w262.

17. MedPAC, "A Path to Bundled Payment."

18. E. S. Fisher, D. E. Wennberg, T. A. Stukel, D. J. Gottlieb, and others, "The Implications of Regional Variations in Medicare Spending. Part 1: The Content, Quality, and Content of Care," *Annals of Internal Medicine* 138 (2003): 273–87; E. S. Fisher, D. E. Wennberg, T. A. Stukel, D. J. Gottlieb, and others, "The Implications of Regional Variations in Medicare Spending. Part 2: Health Outcomes and Satisfaction with Care," *Annals of Internal Medicine* 138 (2003): 288–98.

19. G. Hackbarth, R. Reischauer, and A. Mutti, "Collective Accountability for Medical Care—Toward Bundled Medicare Payments," *New England Journal of Medicine* 359 (2008): 3–5, see p. 5.

20. See the Council of Accountable Physician Practices (CAPP) Web site at http://www.amga-capp.org.

21. R. Gillies, K. Chenok, S. Shortell, G. Pawlson, and others, "The Impact of Health Plan Delivery System Organization on Clinical Quality and Patient Satisfaction," *Health Services Research* 41, no. 4, pt. 1 (2006): 1181–99; W. B. Weeks, D. J. Gottlieb, D. J. Nyweide, J. M. Sutherland, and others, "Do Physician Members of Group Practices Belonging to the Council of Accountable Physician Practices Provide Higher Quality and Lower Cost Health Care to Medicare Beneficiaries Than Their Competitors?" *Health Affairs*, forthcoming.

22. L. Tollen, "Physician Organization in Relation to Quality and Efficiency of Care: A Synthesis of Recent Literature" (New York: The Commonwealth Fund, 2008), http://www.commonwealthfund.org/Content/Publications/Fund-Reports/2008/Apr/Physician-Organization-in-Relation-to-Quality-and-Efficiency-of-Care--A-Synthesis-of-Recent-Literatu.aspx.

23. F. J. Crosson, "The Delivery System Matters," *Health Affairs* 24 (2005): 1543–48.

24. E. S. Fisher, D. O. Staiger, J.P.W. Bynum, and D. J. Gottlieb, "Creating Accountable Care Systems," *Health Affairs* Web exclusive (Dec. 5, 2006), w44–w57, http://content.healthaffairs.org/cgi/reprint/26/1/w44.

25. S. M. Shortell and L. P. Casalino, "Health Care Reform Requires Accountable Care Systems," *JAMA* 30 (2009): 95–7.

26. Fisher and others, "Fostering Accountable Health Care."

27. MedPAC, "Accountable Care Organizations."

28. MedPAC, "Accountable Care Organizations," 43, 56.

29. F. J. Crosson, "Medicare: The Place to Start Delivery System Reform," *Health Affairs* Web exclusive (January 27, 2009), w232–w234, http://content.healthaffairs.org/cgi/reprint/28/2/w232.

30. Fisher and others, "The Implications of Regional Variations in Medicare Spending," Part 1; Fisher and others, "The Implications of Regional Variation in Medicare Spending," Part 2; also see the *Dartmouth Atlas of Health Care* site, http://www.dartmouthatlas.org.

CHAPTER TWO

HISTORY OF PHYSICIAN-HOSPITAL COLLABORATION

Obstacles and Opportunities

Lawton R. Burns
Jeff C. Goldsmith
Ralph W. Muller

Introduction

Management theory teaches that successful innovation requires concomitant changes among the system's components to achieve congruence or *fit*.[1] Similar thinking has been applied to changing the U.S. health care system.[2] In recent years, there has been growing recognition that payment reform of the U.S. health care system must be accompanied by corresponding reforms in the delivery system. Proposed payment models such as bundled payment and gainsharing require new models of physician-hospital relationships to make them work.

Policymakers and researchers who advocate payment reform commonly recognize the need for hospitals and physicians to link together in various organizational models, coordinate their efforts, and achieve three types of integration: economic, clinical, and cultural. Indeed, the Federal Trade Commission (FTC) and Department of Justice (DOJ) have issued guidelines that require providers to demonstrate these different types of integration if they wish to consolidate their practices and jointly negotiate with commercial payers.

Such collaboration is not easy to achieve. For providers, the twentieth century has been characterized as a century of conflict.[3] Much of this conflict stems from the classic problem of trying to integrate professionals into bureaucracies.[4] Such conflict has also been shaped by public and private sector forces specific to the health care industry, forces touching on issues of payment, competition, cost containment, managed care, professional prerogatives, and medical liability.

At the same time, there has been a shift in the relationship between hospitals and physicians throughout the past century. This shift involves the demise of the dual hierarchy of the old hospital (separate medical and administrative spheres), the eclipse of the hospital as the *physicians' workshop*, the rise of corporate forms that envelop physicians, the rise of substantial capital and management support for complex ambulatory practice independent of the hospital, and, at the most general level, the ascendancy of management authority over professional power.

Some of these shifts have occurred with the explicit goal of fostering economic, clinical, or cultural integration in physician-hospital relationships. Nevertheless, it is not clear that integration has changed the care experience in a way that patients and their families actually notice. As a direct consequence, most physician-hospital integration has had limited impact on health care costs or quality.[5] Thus, it is not yet clear whether the ascendancy of management in physician-hospital relationships is beneficial and, if so, in what ways.

This chapter first reviews the changes in physician-hospital relationships across the twentieth century and the industry forces that prompted the arrangements observed. The chapter then argues that the major provider-based competencies called for in health care reform may best be satisfied by hospitals rather than physicians. Despite these advantages, and despite the shift in power to institutions over professionals, hospitals will still encounter problems in collaborating with physicians, and both parties may still encounter problems in working together to improve patient care. Subsequent chapters in this book explore those problems and potential solutions.

Historical Development of Physician-Hospital Relationships

The historical development of physician-hospital relationships necessarily flows from the development of both the hospital industry and the medical profession. The following sections describe these relationships during several major eras in the histories of these two sectors.[6]

1870–1930: The Rise of the Hospital Industry

The rise of the hospital industry took place largely between the years 1870 and 1930 and primarily in the wealthier states and larger cities of the eastern United States.[7] During this period, there were several major technological and therapeutic breakthroughs in medicine, as well as remarkable population increases and economic growth, which together increased demand for hospital services. At the same time, a growing economy and base of philanthropists and trustees supplied the capital to build the infrastructure needed to meet the demand. Although they were historically institutions of care to shelter the poor sponsored by the trustees, hospitals evolved into institutions of cure that attracted wider economic classes of patients. Middle-class (paying) patients were needed to help finance the growing costs of technologically and institutionally based medicine. As Starr writes, the hospital evolved during this period into the physicians' workshop, which the physician both required technologically and controlled economically.

Such an arrangement served physician interests well. Physicians were given access to hospitals and their support staffs without having to deal with managing costs, raising capital, or administering operations—amounting to a huge social subsidy of their private incomes. Physicians were accorded this access in exchange for donating services where needed (for example, taking call in the emergency room, participating on hospital committees) as part of a quid pro quo.

Physician incomes also grew during this period, while hospitals often incurred losses or just broke even. Years later, Clark would criticize hospital tax-exemption as a screen for "for-profit" activities on the part of physicians, who made use of the community's capital on a risk-free and cost-free basis to expand their professional franchises.[8] However, hospitals also benefited from physicians' patronage, because they brought in more paying patients as well as helping the hospital compete with other hospitals being built. This encouraged hospitals to open their medical staffs to community physicians. The majority of physicians had hospital privileges by the end of the period; only a fraction of physicians were either employed or practiced full time in the institution.

Physician access to the institution was coupled with professional autonomy. According to Stevens, nonprofit boards viewed their institutions as valuable instruments of professional expertise and viewed their own roles as supporting rather than controlling that expertise. Trustees thus yielded control over clinical decision making to physicians, who monopolized the scientific knowledge and ability to use the new technologies being developed.[9]

Physician autonomy and control received institutional endorsement in 1912 when the American College of Surgeons (ACS) formed to pursue hospital standardization and again in 1918 when the ACS adopted minimum standards for well-equipped surgical environments. The minimum standards encompassed five quality criteria, including the presence of hospital laboratory and radiology departments under physician supervision.

Hospitals felt compelled to adhere to these requirements for several reasons. Surgery was the central craft in most hospitals. Surgical management was important to reduce infections. The industrial standardization movement begun by Frederick Taylor was well under way. Hospitals also sought to avoid external regulation. As part of the ACS requirements, hospitals had to develop formal medical staff structures, committees, meetings, and policies to supervise standards within the hospital. These requirements were consistent with state hospital licensure statutes, which granted the medical staff semiautonomous status with formal bylaws distinct from the hospital's bylaws.

The hospital was thus assumed to be a physicians' workshop whose clinical affairs were overseen by the medical staff; the physician hierarchy and organization was separate from the administrative hierarchy and organization.[10] Governance arrangements guaranteed physician clinical autonomy, which served both as the bedrock for and constraint on future efforts to improve physician-hospital relationships in the remaining decades of the twentieth century and the beginning of the new century.

Thus, since the early decades of the last century, the American community (or nonteaching) hospital was defined by open access to physicians, use of the hospital as the physicians' workshop, quid pro quo relationships governing the exchange between the hospital and physicians, professional autonomy of the private practitioner, and dual hierarchies of administration and medicine.

In teaching hospitals, by contrast, medical staff membership was tied to faculty appointment in an affiliated medical school or employment by an affiliated university (not necessarily by the hospital). Moreover, there was in these institutions as well an ethical presumption, with legal backing, that faculty physicians would be left alone by the hospital to make patient care decisions.

Stevens does note that a handful of organizational models diverged from the norm: for example, the large private medical groups that directed most of their patients to one hospital. The American Medical Association (AMA) opposed these closed-practice models as the corporate practice of medicine. Likewise, the aforementioned university hospitals were attacked by state medical societies for having closed-staff arrangements. Statements published in the 1930s in the *Journal of the American Medical Association* espoused the profession's key tenets, including solo practice (not group), fee-for-service payment (not salaried), medical professional control of all medical services, and the conviction that medical institutions are but logistical extensions of physician practice.[11]

During this early period, physician-hospital relationships were still occasionally challenged by conflict between the two parties. One source of conflict was hospitals' development of outpatient departments to recruit patients for teaching purposes as "interesting material."[12] Such departments became more critical sources of patients during World War I, when many physicians served in the armed forces, and local physician supply decreased.

Another type of tension was caused by rising hospital expenses and thus rising hospital rates charged to patients. Hospitals expected patients to pay them before the physician was paid. Rapidly rising hospital expenditures meant that a growing share of national health expenditures were now going to institutions (23 percent in 1929) rather than to medical professionals (30 percent).

1930–1965: Third-Party Payment and Dual Hierarchies

The next thirty-five years witnessed major changes in provider payment that strengthened and reaffirmed the principles governing physician-hospital relationships established in the earlier period. At the same time, this era witnessed the rise of several countervailing forces to the professional power of physicians that exacerbated the tensions between hospitals and physicians.

The Great Depression in the 1930s threatened the incomes and survival of both hospitals and physicians. Patients did not have the ability to pay for the care they received from either party. As a result, hospitals were not able to finance the new technologies and therapies being developed. On separate fronts, the hospital industry and the medical profession pushed for a voluntary—rather than a government—solution to health insurance coverage through Blue Cross and Blue Shield plans, respectively. Blue Cross plans needed local physician support to succeed.

Blue Cross plans were careful to not cover physician services or to intertwine hospital with physician payment. Hospitals preserved open staff models for physicians, kept specialist billing separate from the hospital, maintained fee-for-service and physician autonomy, placed physicians in charge of ancillary clinical departments (compensating hospital-based practitioners in a variety of ways), and reaffirmed the hospital's status as the physicians' workshop.

Nevertheless, professional powers were now counterbalanced by several new organizational realities. First, the voluntaristic solution to health insurance coverage traded the possibility of government funding of, and control over, the hospital for local control by the hospital's administration and board.[13] Financial issues, as well as the need to manage the institution's growing operations, required a new class of professionals: hospital administrators. Training programs for this new professional class developed in the 1930s and subsequent decades; professional textbooks and associations followed.

Physicians delegated control over nonclinical functions to this new class, leading to an uneasy balancing of power between the medical and administrative hierarchies.[14] Along with the original hospital founders—the trustees—hospitals now had a triumvirate, or *three-legged stool*, model of governance.[15] Power was shared among the three groups, with conflict avoidance or conflict resolution through growth as two primary ways of muddling through.

Conflicts nevertheless continued to characterize physician-hospital relationships. Starr describes frequent divisions over such issues as further expansions to the hospital's outpatient department, the addition of lay managers to run specialized services, and hospital hiring of full-time physicians to oversee these services. Stevens notes that the major ancillary areas (radiology, pathology, and anesthesiology) had developed powerful technologies and large staffs of nonmedical technicians that the hospital now employed despite their supervision by physicians. These technical staff members heavily outnumbered the physicians in these areas. As the clinical division of labor became more complex, the idea of the hospital as exclusively the physicians' workshop was hard to sustain.

Physician resistance to hospital employment was further exacerbated by the growing number of nonmedical hospital employees who (as in other charitable institutions) were not allowed to unionize under the Wagner Act—a countervailing force to corporate control in other sectors of the economy. Stevens writes that hospitals enjoyed greater control over their workforce for other reasons as well, including their voluntary character and the philanthropy of trustees.[16]

Studies conducted during this period repeatedly cite the management of relationships with physicians as a major problem area for hospital administrators. For example, the 1948 Prall report, which advocated curriculum requirements for university programs of hospital administration, identified physician-hospital relationships as administrators' number one problem.[17] A Cornell University study conducted in 1963 identified these relationships as the number four problem, a finding affirmed in a 1978 study.[18]

According to Stevens, conflicts were natural due to (a) the growing concentration of physicians' practice within the hospital and (b) the lack of clarity of the medical staff's role and authority. Because there was no formal decision-making structure of physicians, administrators lacked a clear party to deal with. Conflicts over issues such as *corporate practice of medicine*, the hospital's involvement in ancillary and outpatient services, and payment of hospital-based practitioners continued to fester. As a result, there was a "smoldering distrust, antagonism, resentment, and even hatred" in physician-hospital relationships.[19]

Two legal rulings at the end of this period chipped away even more at physician autonomy. In 1957 *Bing* v. *Thunig* established hospital liability for contractual relationships with community physicians and responsibility for their behavior inside the institution. In 1965 *Darling* v. *Charleston Community Memorial Hospital* affirmed and extended the hospital's legal responsibility.

Physicians could no longer claim complete freedom from the hospital's jurisdiction; hospitals now had a direct corporate responsibility to supervise the care rendered by physicians within the institution. Hospitals began to ask or demand cooperation from the medical staff for quality assurance. Hospitals also had to exercise care in the selection of physicians who practiced inside and take corrective action when deficient medical practice surfaced. More importantly, these rulings began to establish hospital accountability for patient outcomes.

1965–1990: Medicare and the Consolidation of Hospital Authority

The passage of Medicare and Medicaid in 1965 widened access to health insurance coverage, escalated health care spending, and reaffirmed some historical patterns.[20] Medicare Parts A and B replicated the separate payment silos of hospitals and physicians established under Blue Cross and Blue Shield, respectively, and also outsourced claims management to these private plans. Medicare also continued the practice of fee-for-service reimbursement and free choice of provider, and it explicitly guaranteed clinical autonomy. Medicare was statutorily forbidden to interfere with the practice of medicine.

By the end of the 1960s, some reformers called for concomitant changes in both payment methods and provider organization to cope with the explosive growth in health costs after the enactment of Medicare. These reformers, among them Paul Ellwood, advocated for a model of private group practices affiliated with a primary hospital developed in the 1930s or the emerging prepaid group practice model developed during the 1920s and 1930s on the West Coast. Their objective was to expand the footprint of organizations such as Kaiser Permanente and the Group Health Co-operatives, which combined salaried medical practice and capitated health insurance payment.

The reformers' proposal eventually resulted in new federal legislation, the HMO Act of 1973, signed into law by President Richard Nixon. The provision of federal planning grants enabled medical groups and hospitals to experiment with the creation of new risk-bearing organizations (prepayment plans) coupled with tightly linked physician groups (either employed or contracted) to help manage the risk. There were numerous community-based health plan start-ups, many of which survive to this day. The Marshfield Clinic developed its Community Health Plan in 1971; the Geisinger Clinic and its hospital established its health plan in 1972; the Presbyterian/Lovelace system in Albuquerque established its health plan in 1973; and Michael Reese Hospital in Chicago set up its plan in the early 1970s.

In addition to new payment and provider models, hospitals began to respond to growing challenges by embracing the language of management.

New management structures emerged, such as the investor-owned hospital chains in the late 1960s, which entered the market to take advantage of Medicare's favorable payment model, and to consolidate and strengthen a sector of physician-sponsored hospitals. These chains pioneered horizontal consolidation of facilities, the pursuit of scale economies through more centralized management (for example, centralized support services and supply-chain management), capital fundraising through the equity markets rather than philanthropy, the use of consultants, and the pursuit of efficiency.

Nonprofit hospitals were threatened by the growth of investor-owned hospitals and responded by developing their own regional chains, as well as national purchasing organizations such as the Voluntary Hospitals of America. They also began to access tax-exempt bond markets to finance system-building efforts. Hospitals thus faced the need to keep up with new payment and provider models, new capital financing models, growing Medicare regulation, and the details of Medicare politics. All of these developments served to place even greater power and responsibility with hospital administrators.

Hospitals borrowed ideas of modern management from sources outside the hospital industry as well as inside. Hospitals developed complex corporate structures in which holding companies oversaw a diversified array of businesses, some not even focused on health care. Hospitals also began to develop joint ventures and strategic alliances with one another (for example, through shared services), with their physicians, and with insurers. Hospital administrators and assistant administrators became chief executive officers and chief operating officers. Hospitals began to invest in strategic planning and marketing activities. All of these developments served to transform what used to be a community institution into more of a business enterprise.[21]

Whereas the 1970s was the era of increasing regulation in health care, the 1980s was the era of market forces and market competition. The federal government abandoned the certificate-of-need regulation passed in 1974 and embraced antitrust enforcement and extended it to the health care professions; and many states abandoned the public-utility-style rate regulation of hospitals that was established in the 1970s. Providers' pursuit of management efficiency and the adoption of management strategies were consistent with this new approach. Entrepreneurial efforts, in the form of equity joint ventures and new business models, were similarly encouraged.

The push for modern management reached a high point in 1983 with the passage of a new Medicare Prospective Payment System (PPS) using diagnosis-related groups (DRGs). DRGs reintroduced the idea of standardization first suggested by the ACS reforms of 1918. Rather than standardizing hospital equipment and governance, however, the focus now was on standardizing hospital patterns of treatment. DRGs capped payments for an entire hospitalization, rather than continuing to pay for hospital inpatient services à la carte. This forced hospitals to analyze and then manage care patterns and the intensity of resource use within a hospital stay to avoid ruinous losses under the new payment system. This was impossible without the active support of the medical staff.

Because PPS affected only Part A payments to the hospital, administrators now approached physicians for the first time for their help in operating within a budget constraint—a very stressful moment for both parties. Administrators had an incentive to try to educate physicians about the need for cost containment, to engage them in integrative partnerships such as building joint physician-hospital delivery networks, and to scrutinize physician practice patterns as part of money-making or money-losing services. DRG payment pressures were reinforced by hospital contracting with the burgeoning sector of managed care organizations, which likewise called for hospitals to ask their physicians to work within (some-times capitated) fiscal limits. Private insurers replaced open-ended, after-the-fact "reimbursement" for hospital services with negotiated rates determined in many cases on a per diem or even per case basis.

Physicians were not accustomed to, and thus not quite ready for, such con-versations, which inevitably bred more distrust in their hospital "partners." Hall notes that much of the cost containment effort of the 1980s focused on institu-tional payments (DRG payments to hospitals and capitated payments to health maintenance organizations [HMOs]) because it was more efficient to target and motivate larger organizations than individual professionals.[22] This effort likely had the effect of indirectly motivating institutional control over physicians to limit the institution's risk under these new reimbursement methods.

A new payment methodology for physicians was developed for Medicare Part B in 1992 and implemented in the late 1990s. Physician payment under the resource-based relative value scale (RBRVS) attempted to create a more scientific basis for paying for physician care, but it did not address aligning physicians' financial incentives under Part B more directly with hospitals' incen-tives under Part A.

Hospitals now focused on cost management in their dealings with physicians, reviving old physician complaints about diminished clinical autonomy and the corporate practice of medicine. Hospitals also engaged in *product line management*, often a disguise for cultivating profitable clinical services and jettisoning unprofit-able ones. A decade later, some hospitals would extend this approach from the clinical services to the physician level by imposing *economic credentialing*, evaluating physicians' privileges based in part on their contribution to hospital profit.

Rather than being an open workshop, hospitals began cutting back on some services and uses of technology on campus, while developing networks of remote facilities and services. Hospital forays into the ambulatory care market represented an extension of the outpatient department strategy developed earlier. Hospitals developed freestanding ambulatory services such as imaging, emergency or urgent care, surgery, and rehabilitation and occupational medicine, as well as remote physician office complexes. In some cases, aggressive ambulatory development brought hospitals into direct competition with the community-based physicians on their medical staffs.[23]

At the same time that physicians faced growing incursions from hospitals into their traditional markets, they also faced growing competition from other physicians and other types of practitioners. In response to impending shortages of practitioners, the number of medical schools had expanded, growing from 88 schools in the mid-1960s to 126 schools by 1980. This expansion was encouraged by federal funding for health professions education. Concerns over physician shortages and favorable immigration policies in the 1960s and 1970s also led to growing competition from an influx of international medical graduates, who accounted for nearly one-quarter of all active physicians and filled residency positions by the end of the century.

Finally, as part of the 1970s expansion of homeopathy, osteopathy, and herbal medicine (a return to medicine's nineteenth-century roots), physicians faced growing competition from what are now termed *complementary* and *alternative* medicine practitioners, who increasingly sought membership on the hospital's medical staff. Some physicians blamed the hospital for fomenting part of this new competition. By the 1980s, physicians no longer enjoyed a monopoly over professional services provided to the hospital.

Three legal rulings during this period further exacerbated physician-hospital tensions by increasing the power of hospitals and health plans over physicians. The U.S. Supreme Court, in *Goldfarb* v. *Virginia State Bar* (1975), struck down the learned professions exemption to the Sherman Act—meaning that physicians could now be subject to antitrust scrutiny and charges of restraint of trade in their dealings with hospitals. The 1982 *Arizona* v *Maricopa County Medical Society* decision blocked independent physicians in the Phoenix area from collectively negotiating prices and froze the physician consolidation movement—at a time when hospitals and health plans continued their horizontal integration into local, regional, and national systems.[24]

The resulting uneven playing field gave rise to a growing sense of injustice among physicians and to the growing ability of hospitals to develop local monopolies with leverage over disorganized physicians. In *Jefferson Parish Hospital District No. 2* v. *Hyde* (1984), the U.S. Supreme Court allowed exclusive hospital contracts with specialist physician groups (for example, for coverage of hospital ancillary services). Such contracts did not violate federal antitrust laws, yet they served to block free access to hospital privileges by some community physicians. These contracts prompted several lawsuits brought by excluded physicians and heightened conflict between hospitals and physicians.

Physician-hospital issues were a major reason for the formation of a new section within the AMA: the Hospital Medical Staff Section. This section was formed to help physicians collectively voice their concerns about incursions of the hospital's administration into traditional areas of physician discretion, as well as to create a non-hospital-controlled framework for medical staff leadership development. Three professional associations issued reports in the 1980s emphasizing the growing importance of hospital-physician conflict. These associations included the AMA and the American Hospital Association (AHA),[25] the Joint Commission on Accreditation of Healthcare Organizations (JCAHO),[26] and the AHA's Office of Legal and Regulatory Affairs.[27]

One technique used by hospitals to deal with medical staff conflicts was physician inclusion on the board of trustees (see Chapter Seven). Another was the development of salaried roles such as the chief medical officer and vice president for medical affairs. Hospitals also began to seek alignment or partnerships with segments of the physician community. The physicians thus targeted became customers and feeders to the hospital's outpatient and inpatient service lines.

As the decade drew to a close, the federal Medicare program proposed to include Part B fees of hospital-based specialists (radiologists, pathologists, and anesthesiologists) as part of the inpatient DRGs, effectively capping the Medicare payments for these specialties and giving the hospital explicit control over these income streams. This 1987 proposal was enormously threatening to the independent status and incomes of these powerful specialists, and it engendered sufficient political controversy to be abandoned after widespread congressional opposition.

1990–2009: Managed Care and Market Consolidation

The trends observed during the 1980s accelerated during the 1990s due to several environmental forces. The managed care movement reached its zenith in the mid-1990s, when HMOs penetrated one-third of the large commercially insured market. Such managed care models combined capitated payments with group and staff model clinics, as well as risk-sharing arrangements with physician-based independent practice associations (IPAs).

Capitated plans now included global capitation, in which providers assumed risk for inpatient, outpatient, and sometimes pharmaceutical use and costs. Federal pressures intensified this push to risk sharing in 1993, with the health reform proposals of President Bill Clinton and his wife, Hillary Rodham Clinton. The Clinton plan called for regional health insurance purchasing cooperatives to negotiate with accountable health plans composed of integrated provider networks in local markets.

The rise of HMOs and the threat that the Clinton plan would convert the rest of the provider market into risk-bearing entities induced hospitals and physicians to form a variety of integrated delivery networks. Research shows that 1994 was the modal year for hospitals to develop horizontally integrated networks of hospitals and vertically integrated networks of hospitals and physicians (for example, physician-hospital organizations [PHOs]) and sometimes health plans.[28]

These integrated delivery networks were developed for several purposes. First, they represented a collaborative effort by hospitals and physicians to confront the threat of managed care and develop contracting vehicles for joint bargaining. Hospital consolidation and physician practice acquisition often was explicitly directed at limiting health plan bargaining power. Second, they represented a generic provider response to an uncertain future whose underlying assumptions included closed panel networks, global capitation, and downsizing of provider capacity (number of hospitals, beds, specialists, and so on). All of these assumptions eventually proved to be erroneous. Though the formation of integrated delivery networks accelerated in the early 1990s, it slowed by the end of the decade due to the diminishing number of hospitals yet to be aligned with systems, as well as financial pressures from the Balanced Budget Act of 1997.

It is ironic that strategies that originated in a *procompetition* political environment had explicitly anticompetitive consequences. Hospital consolidation resulted in many metropolitan areas being dominated by a handful of hospital systems that also owned extensive physician practices and related health services. These systems eventually achieved significant bargaining leverage over health plans in the early 2000s.

Consolidation was the mantra of the decade. Nearly every player in the health care value chain—insurers, hospitals, group purchasing organizations, wholesalers, product manufacturers—consolidated its operations through mergers and acquisitions.[29] Integrated delivery networks were a vehicle for providers to pursue this strategy. Such collaborations were initially compelling to physicians because they believed global payments under health reform would be made only to large institutions, not to individual providers, who were constrained from organizing into larger economic units by antitrust laws. In turn, physicians, especially primary care physicians, were now more attractive to hospitals due to the shift to managed care, as hospital systems sought to become sole source contractors with broadly accessible proprietary physician networks.

Hospitals were not the sole consolidators of primary care physician practices. Publicly traded physician practice management (PPM) companies in many markets bid competitively to acquire local practices, seeking to step between hospitals and health plans in risk contract negotiation. Many of these PPM firms did little to improve quality or reduce costs; rather, they were vehicles for executing roll-up strategies designed to quickly build up scale with the hope of garnering managed care contracts and exert bargaining leverage under them.

Research shows that these practice acquisition strategies largely failed to achieve anything, except consume a great deal of hospital and investor capital.[30] The large integrated delivery networks that developed included more levels of bureaucracy, corporate offices separated from the facilities that treated patients, highly paid system executives, greater dependence on expensive external consultants, slower decision making, an emphasis on the front-office mentality over the frontline mentality, little effort to make system changes meaningful to frontline staff, and no real efforts to reduce costs or improve quality.

Health plans found employers reluctant to accept *closed panel* models that relied only on a subset of providers in a given local market. Employees did not want to be forced to switch physicians or hospitals because their employers chose a different health plan. Broad-based health plans, such as preferred provider organizations (PPOs) and point of service (POS) plans, triumphed over closed panel HMO plans. This meant that integrated delivery networks could not offset their development expenses and physician practice acquisition costs and operating losses with additional patient enrollment.

As the 1990s wore on, many health plans wound down capitated contracts and hired disease management firms to carve out troublesome subsets of cost risk—particularly mental health and prescription drugs. New pharmacy benefits management (PBM) firms emerged to manage prescription drug costs, contract with pharmaceutical companies, and impose protocols on health plan members. Health plans also developed their own disease management programs or delegated them to new companies such as COR Solutions and American Healthways. These activities had the effect of bypassing the doctor-patient relationship and attempting to manage cost risk directly.

Many integrated delivery networks experienced both economic and organizational stress, and at least one major bankruptcy ensued from this strategy, that of the Allegheny Health Education and Research Foundation in Pittsburgh and Philadelphia.[31] Despite predictions that they would dominate many health care markets,[32] an entire industry of publicly traded PPM firms such as MedPartners and PhyCor collapsed in less than two years, taking nearly $12 billion in investor equity with them.

The failure of hospital-sponsored primary care physician networks and the PPM companies left a bad taste in physicians' mouths and increased their cynicism and suspicion of the corporate practice of medicine. Despite the rhetoric about *aligned incentives*, these efforts failed to improve physician-hospital relationships. Though some larger systems retained their provider networks, the late 1990s were characterized by dissolution of many physician-hospital contracts. As a result of the failed 1990s experiment with global capitation, few providers (except for isolated IPAs and some group practices) wanted to assume risk.

After this period of divestiture of owned practices, however, hospitals returned to employment of physicians less than a decade later, this time employing specialists as well as primary care physicians. With the impending retirement of the baby boom generation of physicians and falling or stagnant physician incomes, hospital employment offered physicians a buffer from market competition, an avenue to cope with declining skills, and a float until retirement.

Hospitals were not seeking hegemony over physician practice or health plan negotiating leverage in this new wave of practice consolidation. Rather, they responded (in a largely defensive manner) to spreading economic distress in their physician communities. The employment packages developed during the 2000s avoided some of the common mistakes committed during the 1990s, including fewer practice buyouts, less generous compensation packages, shorter income guarantees, and more incentives for clinical productivity and revenue metrics. Still, there is no solid evidence that hospitals have yet learned how to make physician employment profitable; it does not appear to be a core hospital competence.

Two remarkable changes have occurred in the current decade, separating the hospital of the mid-2000s from the hospital of the early 1900s. First, an increasing number of practitioners across the specialty spectrum withdrew from the hospital. More primary care physicians now focus their attention on office-based and ambulatory practice. Many surgical specialists, such as ophthalmologists, urologists, plastic surgeons, and gastroenterologists, have developed completely hospital-independent practices, using freestanding surgical facilities for their practices.

Second, a growing number of physicians are now salaried employees of, or contractors to, the hospital. State medical societies now report that 70 percent to 80 percent of primary care physicians are hospital employees. Hospitals have also begun, with considerable controversy, to employ specialists required to cover the hospital's 24/7 services (such as cardiology and orthopedics). Increasingly, community-based physicians no longer wish to spend time rounding or treating patients in the hospital, and they ask that full-time staff perform these functions at the hospital's expense. Hospitalists, intensivists, laborists, and so on have appeared as full-time employees of the hospital or contractors employed by outside firms or physician groups.

Thus, at the same time as a diminishing percentage of the community's practitioners need to use the hospital, an increasing percentage have become dependent on the hospital for a portion of their incomes. These countervailing forces—the diminished use of the hospital but increasing economic dependency—will create yet new stresses in physician-hospital relationships, as well as exposing hospitals to increasing economic risk.

The 1990s also saw two public sector initiatives to increase care coordination and prepare the economic groundwork for further provider consolidation. First, the Health Care Financing Administration (HCFA, now the Centers for Medicare and Medicaid Services [CMS]) developed the Medicare Participating Heart Bypass Center Demonstration. This program paid a small set of hospitals a bundled payment of Part A and Part B fees for coronary artery bypass graft (CABG) procedures to be split with their physicians. Hospitals participating in the demonstration succeeded in developing new methods of collaborative decision making with their physicians and new approaches to cost containment (see Chapter Five for a case study of one hospital's participation in this program). Nevertheless, HCFA encountered opposition in Congress to extending bundled payment to other procedures, and the demonstration quietly ended. In 2008 CMS announced a return to bundled inpatient payments through the Acute Care Episode Demonstration, which covered an extended set of cardiac and ortho-pedic procedures. In January 2009, CMS announced that five hospitals in the southwestern United States would participate in this new demonstration.

Second, the DOJ and FTC developed antitrust guidelines for combinations of health care firms that would be procompetitive (although some have argued that these guidelines actually provided insufficient guidance to allow firms to act on them—see Chapters One and Six). These guidelines outlined the types of financial or clinical integration that must be present in physician-hospital collaborations and physician networks in order for provider groups legally to engage in collective contracting with managed care organizations. The latter half of the 1990s and the first nine years of the 2000s saw the DOJ and FTC prosecute several provider networks for their failure to adhere to these guidelines.[33] Government agencies prevailed in nearly all of the early prosecutions: physician-hospital associations and IPAs were found to have engaged in price fixing without offering any com-pensatory economic or clinical integration that might lower costs or improve quality. Two exceptions—Advocate HealthCare and Greater Rochester IPA—were allowed to continue based on a demonstrated ability to motivate physicians toward cost and quality goals.

In part to deal with DOJ and FTC requirements and guidance, in part to foster closer relationships with physicians, and in part to generate greater reve-nues, hospitals began to develop an array of noneconomic, economic, and clinical integration arrangements with their physicians. This array has been described elsewhere in the literature.[34] In some cases, hospitals embarked on new strategies such as using proprietary electronic medical record systems to link community physician offices and hospital sites.

In other cases, hospitals revisited older strategies and repackaged them under new names such as *hospital service lines* (formerly *product lines*). As in the 1980s with DRGs, hospitals pursued growth of those service lines that were "winners" (specialty areas such as cardiology, orthopedics, neurosurgery, and oncology), or that generated significant revenues and margins for the hospital. This approach served to divide the medical staff into "home run" physicians versus "singles" physicians, as well as to divide the various specialties into fiefdoms with physician service line chiefs as their feudal lords.

Another development of the 2000s further segmented physician markets. Specialists in a given community began to aggregate into large single-specialty medical groups to gain bargaining leverage with managed care organizations. This strategy was particularly popular with technology-dependent specialists such as radiologists, urologists, gastroenterologists, and cardiologists, who could not only leverage their bargaining power with health plans but acquire their own imaging equipment under the in-office ancillary service exemption to the Stark laws concerning self-referral (see below and Chapter Six). Such groups have faced growing scrutiny by the DOJ and FTC. These governmental bodies have looked for economic and clinical integration benefits to justify the higher reimbursement that the groups have sought from payers.

The development of large single-specialty groups ran against the grain of the integrated, multidisciplinary clinics such as Kaiser Permanente, Mayo, and Geisinger, which were held out by policymakers as exemplars of how physicians ought to consolidate. Unfortunately, large multispecialty clinics (100-plus physicians) represent only 1 percent of all group practices, leaving few such practices upon which to build new Kaisers and Mayos.[35] Today, single-specialty groups constitute the single largest block of group practices. Their formation did not solve many problems faced in physician-hospital relationships but rather served as a vehicle for stripping away ancillary services that contributed significant hospital profits. These groups also leveraged their bargaining power to demand subsidies from the hospital for performing hospital-related services, such as covering emergency room call.[36]

Investor-owned companies such as MedCath encouraged physician entrepreneurial efforts by taking on "profitable" physicians such as cardiologists and orthopedic surgeons directly as investors in their hospitals. Surgeons also invested in such facilities, as well as freestanding surgical centers, to augment their incomes and capture a portion of the facility fees generated by moving their patients.

The facilities served as new competitors for hospitals, particularly the smaller community hospitals that depended more heavily on outpatient surgical volumes and lower-severity patients. McKinsey recently estimated that physician dividends from partnerships with ambulatory surgical and imaging companies amounted to $8 billion in 2006.[37]

At the same time, the spread of physician-owned ambulatory surgery centers and office-based surgery and imaging continued the long-standing duel between hospitals and physicians for control over outpatient services, while the freestanding specialty hospitals threatened to strip away from general hospitals the more profitable and lower-severity inpatient cases. These developments directly threatened the core profitability of hospitals, which was increasingly focused in elective outpatient care. McKinsey estimated that a remarkable 75 percent of hospital profits in 2008 came from elective outpatient care, and only 12 percent from inpatient hospitalization.[38] Hospitals threatened by these potential competitors often felt compelled to create physician joint ventures that helped retain some of their profitable outpatient volume and keep physicians from leaving the hospital campus (at the price of giving away half or more of those services' profits).

In addition, pharmaceutical and medical device companies developed an array of financial arrangements—real or sham consulting agreements, "lecture fees," and so on—that sometimes constituted thinly disguised bribes to both primary care physicians and specialists. These economic inducements sought to lock in physician use of their products and prevent hospitals or PBM firms from achieving bargaining leverage through group purchasing that would have lowered manufacturer margins. Such arrangements, struck by firms with very deep pockets and aimed at influential physicians whose incomes had stagnated, also served further to divide physicians from their hospitals.[39]

To respond to the flourishing *moral hazard* opportunities created by physician ownership or control of lucrative technology, the Omnibus Budget Reconciliation Acts of 1989 and 1993 included the famous Stark laws, which forbade physicians from profiting from self-referral of Medicare patients to facilities or services they owned. These laws were riddled with loopholes, however. The most controversial safe harbors for physicians were exemptions for ownership of entire hospitals (as opposed to a specialty center within a hospital) and referral to so-called ancillary services in physicians' own offices, which applied not only to group practices but to technology housed in their office buildings and even to individual physicians who purchased their own computed tomography (CT) or magnetic resonance imaging (MRI) scanners.

The Stark laws marked the beginning of efforts to clamp down on physician self-referrals and business development.[40] They led to a wave of consolidation in the imaging center business, as imaging centers that relied on physician partnerships were forced to restructure their business arrangements and consolidated into two large firms. When the Balanced Budget Act of 1997 brought reductions in payments for imaging services, these companies, in turn, ran into economic difficulties and were forced into bankruptcy.[41]

A new cycle of consolidation was launched in 2005 when the Deficit Reduction Act reduced payments to freestanding imaging facilities for high-technology scans such as MRI and CT, and in 2007 when CMS decided to reduce payments to freestanding ambulatory surgery centers to 65 percent of the fees paid to hospital outpatient departments. It is still too early to tell how significant an effect these changes have had, but radiologists who relied extensively on technical component (or facilities) income as opposed to professional fee income saw significant reductions in their incomes from the Deficit Reduction Act.[42] These changes had the effect of tilting the playing field back in the direction of hospital-sponsored ambulatory services, whose payment levels were not affected.

Overall, the entrepreneurial efforts of physicians seem to have come up short. During the early 2000s, CMS imposed a temporary moratorium on the development of new specialty hospitals, pending an analysis of their performance effects and impact on general hospitals. That analysis showed that these hospitals cream-skimmed patients and did not offer lower-cost, higher-quality care.[43] However, there was also no significant impact on the financial health of general hospitals. The evidence for physician-owned ambulatory surgery centers paralleled these findings.[44]

It is possible that further restrictions on physician entrepreneurship will be included in health reform legislation. A recent article in the *New Yorker* magazine, by Atul Gawande, shined a harsh light on a single Texas community where physician entrepreneurship appears to have dramatically affected Medicare spending in the area.[45] The negative climate developing around physician entrepreneurship may motivate even more risk avoidance among physicians and lead them to seek hospital employment and other relationships.

However, as physicians' income growth has faltered so has the formerly voluntary compact with hospitals under which physicians traded medical staff privileges for covering medical service needs of patients after hours and on weekends. These demands are particularly acute for surgical coverage of the emergency room and coverage of the intensive care units that operate twenty-four hours a day, seven days a week. As fewer physicians, particularly procedure-oriented physicians, need to use the hospital, physicians in critical care disciplines demand and receive stipends for covering call, dramatically increasing hospital costs.[46]

The situation differs in the larger academic medical centers (see Chapter Ten). Their medical staffs consist of a group of physicians—the clinical faculty of the affiliated medical school—employed by the parent university rather than by the hospital. Depending on the institution, these staffs may or may not be organized in the manner of large multispecialty groups; at a minimum, they do aggregate physician billing and payer-bargaining functions. As employees, physicians are protected from the day-to-day productivity requirements of the medical practice market.[47] Being organized in practice plans, faculty physicians can usually negotiate together with the hospital for better payments in the commercial insurance market; teaching hospitals also receive enhanced Medicare payments and, in many states, better payments from the state Medicaid program.

Medical schools often receive significant additional subsidies from their affiliated hospitals in exchange for faculty supervision, which cannot be billed directly to Medicare or other payers. Finally, because they are organized under common governance, these hospitals and faculty practice plans are able to share revenues through means such as gainsharing that avoid some of the conflicts that community hospitals face when physicians split off profitable practices from the hospital (for example, ambulatory surgery centers and imaging facilities) as a means to access facility payments (for example, Medicare Part A or Part B technical).[48]

2010 and Beyond

By the end of the first decade of the 2000s, physicians appear to have lost the battle to retain their autonomy from the hospital and maintain the professional prerogatives developed one hundred years earlier. However, because their practices are, traditionally, small economic units and fragmented along specialty lines, physicians have also failed to organize themselves effectively. They have also been actively inhibited from doing so by federal antitrust law.

Medical staff organizations consist of a confusing matrix of officers, committees, and departments with no strong, central leadership or clear lines of authority. In larger institutions, at least, real power lies in the specialty departments and their chiefs. Hospitals are left with the responsibility to organize physicians and work out patterns of collaboration within and across specialties (service lines, collaborative care models) and distribution of shared fees (bundled payments) and shared savings (gainsharing).

At the same time, physicians have become increasingly dependent on the hospital for incremental income. As baby boom primary care physicians retire, their practices are increasingly absorbed into the hospital, and new primary care physicians become hospital employees. Dependence is evident from the gradual demise of solo practice,[49] the rise in hospital employment, the use of productivity systems to reward employed physicians for their inpatient work, and an increasing emphasis on physicians' production of relative value units in their clinical practice. The physicians' workshop is evolving by degrees into more of a hospital sweatshop (or at least a hospital dependency).

Community-based physician groups are also becoming more reliant on the hospital to help recruit and finance new members. Many specialty groups found their practices did not throw off enough cash flow to replace existing practitioners, and they turned to hospitals for subsidies to maintain their current physician complements. Hospitals witnessed rising levels of admissions from the emergency department (upward of 40 percent in many institutions) not directed by any community practice. These patients were increasingly managed by hospitalists, who were hospital employees or contractors. Thus an increasing fraction of the hospital's admissions and costs are no longer controlled or even affected by community physicians.

These trends are being reinforced by generational changes taking place within the medical profession. As Goldsmith has noted, as the 1960s generation of physicians began to gear down their practices or retire, many have sought hospital employment as either salaried practitioners or medical staff officers.[50] Younger physicians are more diverse along racial, ethnic, and (especially) gender lines. The growing number of younger and female physicians desire more balance between professional and private lives, fewer hours, and more shift work. An increasing percentage of the physician workforce wishes to work part time.

However, younger physicians benchmark their income expectations based on the eighty-hour-a-week work norms of the older physicians they are replacing, placing the hospital in a difficult economic position. They also raise complex questions of equity—whether the hospital is dealing in an aboveboard and evenhanded fashion with physicians who are not receiving economic subsidies or are not employed by the hospital—the very issues that caused so much grief during the 1990s.

The Hospital's Growing Responsibility for Clinical Risk and Cost

The current policy environment in health care may compel major changes in how providers are paid and organized. These new (or not so new) ideas all have a common theme: the expansion of the hospital's responsibility for clinical risk and costs that the hospital cannot manage without active physician collaboration. They will require fundamental changes in how physicians and hospitals collaborate in making decisions, even as the physician community fragments and fewer physicians use the hospital on a daily basis.

As described in Chapters Three and Four, new or proposed payment methodologies will require hospitals and physicians to work together in ways for which they have little historical preparation or a poor historical track record.[51] *Accountable care organizations* (ACOs), described in Chapter Three, call for providers in a wide geographic catchment area to be clinically and fiscally accountable for the entire continuum of care that patients may need. *Bundled payments* likely require providers to coordinate care and distribute payments across all of the in-house specialties involved in a surgical procedure (for example, cardiovascular and orthopedic), or across various types of providers over time. *Pay-for-performance* in the hospital setting requires providers to convene specialists and ancillary staff across many departments to reduce infection rates and other categories of clinical risk. *Incentive payments for reduced readmissions* require providers to improve discharge planning and community-based follow-up of patients. *Incentive payments for clinical integration* require providers to invest in (among other things) electronic medical record systems and implementation spanning inpatient areas, outpatient areas, and community physician offices. Finally, growing calls for *comparative clinical effectiveness* will require providers to screen and evaluate more carefully the new technologies being brought into the hospital by physician advocates and product sales representatives on both quality and cost criteria.

By virtue of their fragmented and silo-based practice organization, the constraints placed on entrepreneurship, their lack of access to capital, and increasing isolation from hospital practice, physicians in many communities are not well organized to accomplish these tasks and may not be inclined to take them on. Just as most physicians shied away from running their own hospitals at the beginning of the twentieth century and delegated these tasks to administrators, many contemporary physicians may prefer that lay managers attempt to organize responses to these new demands for collaboration.

Subsequent chapters provide examples of where physician-led entities have assumed these responsibilities. With the exception of some physician-led organizations (for example, Kaiser Permanente and Mayo Clinic), however, calls for improved care coordination and accountability for cost and quality may be answered more effectively by hospitals, their managers, and their paid clinical directors. As organizations used to being regulated and accredited, hospitals and their managerial cadre have some structural advantage over less-organized physicians in the majority of practice settings in coordinating multiple clinical services, developing models of multidisciplinary care, taking accountability for outcomes, developing care networks, assuming economic risk, managing large provider organizations, managing bundled payments, and doing technology assessments.

This comparative advantage does not necessarily translate into actual competence, however. Hospital and system executives still face a steep learning curve themselves, particularly after the sobering and costly failures of the 1990s.

The present situation thus presents both the opportunity for greater collaboration between hospitals and physicians and challenges in fostering good relationships. In contrast to the early historical dominance of physicians and then the later uneasy balance of power between physicians and hospitals, hospitals now appear to have a constitutional and functional advantage in being organized.

Research on mergers and acquisitions in industry shows that mergers of equally large and powerful firms have difficulty in resolving the difficult political issues of "who is in charge" and "who is being acquired by whom."[52] In such mergers, the extraordinary efforts needed to manage the politics and conflicts of integration drain the energies needed to extract synergies from the combination. Here, however, what is being contemplated is not a merger between like organizations, but rather between a solid and a gas, that is, between a hospital organization and an amorphous *medical community* that has been dispersed both geographically and economically.

These problems were illustrated by the experiences of the 1990s movement toward integrated delivery networks, when hospitals developed a menu of alignment options for physicians (for example, PHO, IPA) who did not necessarily want full integration with the hospital (in other words, employment). Such pluralistic alignment models were almost always failures (with an occasional success story).[53] These failures should chasten advocates of joint physician-hospital risk management, including some of the models that have been called accountable care organizations, which appear to be a reemergence of a troubled 1990s idea, the physician-hospital organization (PHO).

The only alignment model from the 1990s that appears to have persevered and developed is the employment model. Hospitals that retained their employed physicians from this period have spent the ensuing decade attempting to meld acquired practices into a coherent clinical enterprise, with the capabilities of established multispecialty medical groups. How many have actually achieved this coherence will be a subject of future health services research interest.

Thus, from a mergers and acquisitions perspective, the current asymmetry in power between hospitals and physicians might bode well for extracting value from relationships between hospitals and physicians, because it might lessen the political struggle over who is in charge. This is not meant to suggest that asymmetry in power, rather than power sharing through common incentives, is the desired goal. However, the history of physician-hospital relationships described in this chapter evinces persistent, longstanding conflicts between the two parties that inhibit power sharing and common incentives. These conflicts include hospital incursions into outpatient care, control over referrals to the hospital medical staff, control over the technology base in the hospital (and who generates monies from it), physician concerns over commingled reimbursement, physicians' concerns over hospital domination and control (especially through employment relationships), physician concerns over the corporate practice of medicine, and conflicts over covering call for emergency patients. Such conflicts are not likely to disappear quickly, but may attenuate as new generations of physicians replace older generations.

Managing physician-hospital relationships is likely to continue to be a key priority among hospital executives, as it has been since the 1940s. The management skills required here include bargaining and negotiation, conflict resolution, interdisciplinary team building, physician leadership development, management infrastructure development, communication, managing professional-bureaucracy relationships, managing "stars," as well as managing coalitions and politics. Such skills are not well taught in health administration programs and are only recent additions to the curricula of many business schools.

Conclusion

Those responsible for managing physician-hospital relationships might also consider new opportunities for hospitals to add value to their physicians' practices. One major opportunity is improving physician cash flow.[54] Hospitals should invest in digital real-time systems for processing physician billing and collections, and invest in upgrading office systems and staffing to enable better operations.

A second opportunity is developing physician teamwork and collegiality (for example, through executive education and colocation of specialists). These are the features that distinguish and unite physicians at Kaiser Permanente, Mayo, and Geisinger—not how they are paid or who owns what (issues that themselves took generations to resolve at these organizations). According to Freidson, collegiality is also how physicians control the quality of each other's work and thereby minimize the need for outside surveillance and interference.[55] Collegiality also addresses the principal challenge of uniting a physician network: the political struggle of coordinating different specialties with different needs, including renewed attention to professionalism.

Professionalism is also fostered by regulatory oversight of conflict of interest behaviors by physicians (for example, payments from device manufacturers, self-referral, and so on). External oversight may spur greater provider efforts at self-policing of behaviors. Other areas of opportunity include using clinical information systems to develop online clinical communities, assisting primary care physicians and specialists with quality improvement activities as they adapt to pay-for-performance incentives, helping the medical staff to reorganize itself and reengineer its processes, and helping primary care physicians develop new operational models.

The regulatory focus of the Obama administration, compared to the market orientation of the previous Bush administration, will push more physicians into relationships with hospitals. What will these look like? Can hospitals and their managers develop the skills, leadership, and organizational capacity to manage all these conflicting crosscurrents? There will probably be more restrictions on physician self-referral, conflicts of interest that compromise the physician-patient relationship, physician entrepreneurial activities that drive up costs, medical practices that are not cost effective, and capital investments by physicians. It is not clear whether and how physicians will respond to these developments.

It is also unclear whether hospitals' differential ability to handle the potential changes identified in this chapter will help to improve health care's cost and quality issues. In the past, hospitals have relied heavily on structural mechanisms to collaborate with physicians: salaried employment, leadership roles, contracting vehicles, modes of integration, and so on. There is little solid evidence that the use of these mechanisms in hospital settings has helped the pursuit of value. Hospitals might consider other approaches in the future, such as behavioral change skills and rules-based integration.

The next decade of physician-hospital relationships appears to be fraught with new challenges and opportunities to improve the quality of clinical medicine. These challenges will take the form of real and perceived legal barriers, differences in culture between hospitals and physicians (and among physicians), and major differences in governance structures, among others. Each of these topics is explored further in the chapters that follow.

Notes

1. M. L. Tushman and C. A. O'Reilly, *Winning Through Innovation* (Boston: Harvard Business, 1997).

2. Institute of Medicine, *Crossing the Quality Chasm: A New Health System for the 21st Century* (Washington, D.C.: National Academies Press, 2001).

3. P. M. Starr, *The Social Transformation of American Medicine* (New York: Basic Books, 1982); R. Stevens, *In Sickness and in Wealth: American Hospitals in the Twentieth Century* (New York: Basic Books, 1989).

4. R. K. Merton, *Social Theory and Social Structure* (New York: Free Press, 1957); E. Freidson, *The Profession of Medicine* (New York: HarperCollins, 1970); A. Abbott, *The System of Professions* (Chicago: University of Chicago Press, 1988); J. W. Lorsch and T. J. Tierney, *Aligning the Stars* (Boston: Harvard Business, 2002).

5. L. R. Burns and R. W. Muller, "Hospital-Physician Collaboration: Landscape of Economic Integration and Impact on Clinical Integration," *Milbank Quarterly* 86, no. 3 (2008): 375–434.

6. This section and the next rely heavily on historical material reported by P. M. Starr, *The Social Transformation of American Medicine*, and especially R. Stevens, *In Sickness and in Wealth*. Rather than cite these works repeatedly, we are acknowledging them up front.

7. The Hill-Burton Act of 1946 extended federal funding for hospital construction in the South, poorer states, and smaller cities. Much of that development occurred in the 1950s and 1960s.

8. R. C. Clark, "Does the Not-for-Profit Form Fit the Hospital Industry?" *Harvard Law Review* 93, no. 73 (1980): 1416–89.

9. C. Perrow, "Goals and Power Structures," in *The Hospital in Modern Society*, ed. E. Freidson, 112–46 (New York: Free Press, 1963).

10. M. V. Pauly and M. Redisch, "The Not-for-Profit Hospital as a Physicians' Cooperative," *American Economic Review* 63, no. 1 (1973): 87–100; J. F. Harris, "The Internal Organization of Hospitals: Some Economic Implications," *Bell Journal of Economics* 8, no. 2 (1978): 467–82.

11. "Minutes of the Eighty-Fifth Annual Session of the American Medical Association, Held at Cleveland, June 11–15, 1934," *JAMA* 102, no. 26 (1934): 2191–2207.

12. Stevens, *In Sickness and in Wealth*, 87.

13. Stevens, *In Sickness and in Wealth*, chaps. 6 and 7.

14. Perrow, "Goals and Power Structures."

15. R. L. Johnson, "Revisiting 'the Wobbly Three-Legged Stool,'" *Health Care Management Review* 4 (1979): 15–22.

16. Stevens, *In Sickness and in Wealth*, 180.

17. C. Prall, *Problems of Hospital Administration* (Chicago: Physicians' Record Co., 1948).

18. M. T. Dolson, "How Administrators Rate Different Tasks," *Modern Hospital* 7 (1965): 94–97, 166; W. B. Carper, "A Longitudinal Analysis of the Problems of Hospital Administrators," *Hospital and Health Services Administration* 27 (1982): 82–95.

19. Stevens, *In Sickness and in Wealth*, 244.

20. This chapter section and the next draw heavily on J. Goldsmith's many essays on physicians and physician-hospital relationships written over the last thirty years. These include the following articles, arranged alphabetically by article title: "Burning the Seed Corn," *Healthcare Forum Journal* (March/April 1996): 19–22; "The Changing of the Guard: Implications for Hospitals," *Healthcare Strategy Alert* no. 4 (2008): 12–13; "Driving the Nitroglycerine Truck," *Healthcare Forum Journal* (March/April 1993): 36–44; "Farewell to the Voluntary Fireman," *Harvard Business Review* (May/June 1979): 17–18; "Hospitals and Physicians: Not a Pretty Picture," *Health Affairs* Web exclusive (Dec. 5, 2006): w72–w75, http://content.healthaffairs.org/cgi/content/abstract/26/1/w72; "The Illusive Logic of Integration," *Healthcare Forum Journal* (September/October 1994): 26–31; "Integration Reconsidered: Five Strategies for Improved Performance," *Health Care Strategist* (November 1998): 1–8; "M.D.s Deny, Finally Accept Change," *Modern Healthcare* (January 1984): 108–110; "Visions of Empire: Some Problems with the Corporate Model of Physicians," *Hospital Forum* (May/June 1985): 50–52.

21. L. R. Burns, "The Transformation of the American Hospital: From Community Institution Towards Business Enterprise," in *Comparative Social Research*, vol. 12: *Business Institutions*, ed. C. Calhoun, 77–112 (Greenwich, CT: JAI Press, 1990).

22. M. A. Hall, "Institutional Control of Physician Behavior: Legal Barriers to Health Care Cost Containment," *University of Pennsylvania Law Review* 137 (1988): 431–546.

23. Hospital ambulatory development directed capital into areas not subject to the cost limits of inpatient DRGs, but also capitalized on the growing use of less-invasive surgical and diagnostic technologies, which gained momentum during the 1980s.

24. Technically, this decision affected the balance of power between physicians and health plans but not between physicians and hospitals.

25. American Medical Association (AMA) and American Hospital Association (AHA), *The Report of the Joint Task Force on Hospital-Medical Staff Relationships* (Chicago: AMA and AHA, 1985).

26. Joint Commission on Accreditation of Healthcare Organizations (JCAHO), *Report on the Joint Commission Survey of Relationships Among Governing Bodies, Management, and Medical Staffs in U.S. Hospitals* (Chicago: JCAHO, 1988).

27. AHA, *The Report of the Task Force on Dispute Resolution in Hospital-Medical Staff Relationships* (Chicago: AHA, 1988).

28. L. R. Burns, G. Gimm, and S. Nicholson, "The Financial Performance of Integrated Health Organizations (IHOs)," *Journal of Healthcare Management* 50, no. 3 (2005): 191–213.

29. L. R. Burns and D. R. Wholey, "Responding to a Consolidating Healthcare System: Options for Physician Organizations," in *Advances in Health Care Management*, vol. 1, ed. J. Blair, M. Fottler, and G. Savage, 273–335 (New York: Elsevier, 2000).

30. U. Reinhardt, "The Rise and Fall of the Physician Practice Management Industry," *Health Affairs* 19, no. 1 (2000): 42–55; L. R. Burns and M. V. Pauly, "Integrated Delivery Networks (IDNs): A Detour on the Road to Integrated Healthcare?" *Health Affairs* 21, no. 4 (2002): 128–43.

31. L. R. Burns, J. Cacciamani, J. Clement, and W. Aquino, "The Fall of the House of AHERF: The Allegheny Bankruptcy," *Health Affairs* 19, no. 1 (2000): 7–41.

32. J. C. Robinson, "Financial Capital and Intellectual Capital in Physician Practice Management," *Health Affairs* 17, no. 4 (1998): 53–74.

33. L. Casalino, "The Federal Trade Commission, Clinical Integration, and the Organization of Physician Practice," *Journal of Health Politics, Policy and Law* 31, no. 3 (2006): 569–86.

34. Burns and Muller, "Hospital-Physician Collaboration."

35. L. R. Burns, "Perspectives on Physician Group Practices," testimony to MedPAC, Washington, D.C., October 2006; AMA, *Medical Group Practices in the U.S., 2006 Edition* (Chicago: AMA, 2006).

36. Confronted by the prevalence and growth of single-specialty groups, the hospital had no one to turn to who could speak for all specialties or assume accountability for care. Such networks could not work out collaborative agreements with specialist networks in other clinical areas. They also could not take a system focus. These single-specialty groups developed independently of the hospital. However, they potentially served as new contracting partners for hospitals that wanted to outsource management of hospital specialty and ancillary areas to organized provider groups. Such groups may not want to assume accountability for clinical outcomes, given the fact that they were assembled for economic reasons and typically invested little in clinical integration activities. However, the opportunity exists for forging closer hospital ties and assuming more clinical accountability in order for them to get the contracts to manage the hospital's specialty areas.

37. D. Farrell, E. Jensen, B. Kocher, and others, *Accounting for the Cost of U.S. Health Care: A New Look at Why Americans Spend More* (New York: McKinsey Global Institute, December 2008), p. 15.

38. Farrell and others, *Accounting for the Cost of U.S. Health Care.*

39. L. R. Burns, D. Nash, and D. R. Wholey, "The Evolving Role of Third Parties in the Hospital-Physician Relationship," *American Journal of Medical Quality* 22, no. 6 (2007): 402–9.

40. Within the last few years, the Department of Justice has investigated the payments made by medical device manufacturers to orthopedic surgeons (sometimes as inducements to use their implants) and required such payments to be posted on the Internet. Such payments have the effect of dividing physicians from hospitals and aligning them more closely with manufacturers (see Burns, Nash, and Wholey, "The Evolving Role of Third Parties").

41. J. Burklund, "Historical Review of Mergers and Acquisitions in Diagnostic Imaging,"*Radiology Business Journal* (Winter 2008): 44–47.

42. J. W. Moser and D. M. Hastreiter, "2007 Survey of Radiologists: Source of Income and Impact of the Deficit Reduction Act of 2005," *Journal of the American College of Radiology* 6, no. 6 (2009): 408–16.

43. A. Tynan, E. November, J. Lauer, H. Pham, and others, "General Hospitals, Specialty Hospitals and Financially Vulnerable Patients" (Center for Studying Health System Change Research Brief no. 11, April 2009), http://www.hschange.com/CONTENT/1056; K. Carey, J. F. Burgess, and G. J. Young, "Specialty and Full-Service Hospitals: A Comparative Cost Analysis," *Health Services Research* 43, pt. 2 (2008): 1869–87.

44. A. S. Chukmaitov, N. Menachemi, L. S. Brown, C. Saunders, and others, "A Comparative Study of Quality Outcomes in Freestanding Ambulatory Surgery Centers and Hospital-Based Outpatient Departments: 1997–2004," *Health Services Research* 43, no. 5 (2008): 1485–1504; A. Winter, "Comparing the Mix of Patients in Various Outpatient Surgery Settings," *Health Affairs* 22, no. 6 (2003): 68–75; L. P. Casalino, K. J. Devers, and L. R. Brewster, "Focused Factories? Physician-Owned Specialty Hospitals," *Health Affairs* 22 (2003): 56–67.

45. A. Gawande, "The Cost Conundrum: What a Texas Town Can Teach Us About Health Care," *New Yorker,* June 1, 2009, 36–44.

46. Goldsmith, "Hospitals and Physicians: Not a Pretty Picture."

47. At the same time, however, many of these faculty practice plans are specialty dominated and function more as collections of specialty practices than as clinically integrated groups like Mayo or Geisinger.

48. The financial margins of teaching hospitals provide direct support of the research and teaching missions of the university, thereby creating a cross-subsidy of valuable public activity that enhances their community standing and regard. These teaching hospitals are powerful economic actors and often are among the largest employers in their communities, as well as the largest provider of care.

49. S. L. Isaacs, P. S. Jellinek, and W. L. Ray, "The Independent Physician—Going, Going . . . " *New England Journal of Medicine* 360 (2009): 655–57.

50. Goldsmith, "The Changing of the Guard."

51. *Medical homes* call for primary care physicians to coordinate patient services and referrals across a wide network of specialists but not with hospitals.

52. H. Singh, "Big Deal(s): What's Driving the M&A Frenzy?" Knowledge@Wharton (January 24, 2007), http://knowledge.wharton.upenn.edu/article.cfm?articleid=1647 (accessed December 14, 2009).

53. Burns and Pauly, "Integrated Delivery Networks (IDNs)"; Burns and Muller, "Hospital-Physician Collaboration"; L. R. Burns and D. P. Thorpe, "Physician-Hospital Organizations: Strategy, Structure, and Conduct," in *Integrating the Practice of Medicine*, ed. R. Conners, 351–71 (Chicago: AHA, 1997); L. R. Burns and D. R. Wholey. "Responding to a Consolidating Healthcare System."
54. Burns and Muller, "Hospital-Physician Collaboration."
55. E. Freidson, *Doctoring Together* (Chicago: University of Chicago Press, 1975).

CHAPTER THREE

ACHIEVING THE VISION

Structural Change

Stephen M. Shortell
Lawrence P. Casalino
Elliott S. Fisher

Introduction

Americans spend the majority of their health care resources on hospitals and physicians—approximately 60 percent of all health care expenditures are for these services. In a system that is widely recognized to be unsustainable and whose quality is at best uneven, hospitals and physicians are central players in improving a delivery system that has broad and deep effects on the American economy. This will require a fundamental reexamination of how hospitals and physicians do their work. As the opening chapter of this book indicates, this will be a difficult task.

Over the last twenty years, research has highlighted the marked variations across both regions and health systems in patterns of treatment and the overall costs of care for Medicare beneficiaries.[1] Most of the differences in spending are due to greater use of the hospital as a site of care, more frequent referrals to specialists, and greater use of ancillary services such as imaging services or minor tests.[2] The local supply of specialists and hospital resources explains some of the difference in utilization across regions,[3] but physicians' propensity toward a more interventional practice, especially in settings where clinical judgment is required, appears to play a particularly important role.[4] The evidence that higher spending and higher-intensity practice are associated with lower quality and equal or worse health outcomes compared to less spending and intensity has raised the possibility of substantial improvement in the overall efficiency of the U.S. health care system.[5]

The Institute of Medicine and others have pointed to a number of factors that contribute to the relative inefficiency of U.S. health care, including the high degree of fragmentation of the current delivery system; a payment system that reinforces this fragmentation and rewards growth and increased utilization, whether services are beneficial or not; and, lack of shared accountability among providers for coordination, quality and the overall costs of care for the population they serve.[6] The need to bring together providers—especially hospitals and physicians—has led many to call for the development of organizations that can be held more accountable for the full continuum of patients' care.[7]

This chapter addresses that challenge by suggesting different models for organizing the delivery of health care services that have the potential to achieve greater alignment and integration between hospitals and physicians. *Alignment* refers to the condition of close cooperation between two or more parties. *Integration* refers to bringing different parties together into a unified whole. The models proposed provide examples of both alignment and integration.

As highlighted by the Institute of Medicine and underscored in Chapter One of this book, the goals of the health care system are to provide care that is safe, effective, efficient, personalized, timely, and equitable. We currently fall far short of consistently producing these desired outcomes. As shown in Figure 3.1, care systems are needed in which the component organizations facilitate the work of high-performing, patient-centered teams. This will require these care systems to address six key redesign challenges:

- Implementing clinical care processes using guidelines, pathways, protocols, checklists, and related tools
- Making effective use of new electronic information technology
- Capturing and sharing the explosion of new medical knowledge and skills
- Developing effective teams
- Coordinating care across multiple conditions, providers, and settings over time
- Using performance and outcomes measures for both internal quality improvement and external accountability

The stark realization is that, with few exceptions, most hospitals and physicians are simply incapable of doing this work. They are not organized to do so. The task is made more difficult, of course, by a largely toxic payment and regulatory

FIGURE 3.1   MAKING CHANGE POSSIBLE

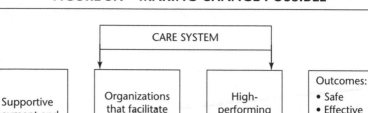

CARE SYSTEM

| Supportive payment and regulatory environment | → | Organizations that facilitate the work of patient-centered teams | → | High-performing patient-centered teams | → | Outcomes:
• Safe
• Effective
• Efficient
• Personalized
• Timely
• Equitable |

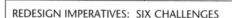

REDESIGN IMPERATIVES: SIX CHALLENGES

- Redesigned care processes
- Effective use of information technologies
- Knowledge and skills management
- Development of effective teams
- Coordination of care across patient conditions, services, and settings over time
- Use of performance and outcome measurement for continuous quality improvement and accountability

Source: Institute of Medicine, *Crossing the Quality Chasm: A New Health System for the 21st Century* (Washington, D.C., National Academies Press, 2001), p. 127. Reprinted with permission from the National Academies Press, Copyright 2010, National Academy of Sciences.

environment (see the far left box in Figure 3.1 and Chapter Four) that frequently creates disincentives for redesigning the delivery process.

The sections that follow highlight the challenge of hospital-physician integration and alignment and provide some organizational arrangements for bringing hospitals and physicians closer together. These models, when combined with a more supportive payment and regulatory environment and greater transparency, may be better able to provide care that is more safe, effective, efficient, personalized, timely, and equitable than the care Americans now receive. The challenges inherent in physician-hospital relationships are discussed first. The concept of the accountable care organization is then introduced; such organizations offer a means to better align the interests of hospitals and physicians. Four distinct organizational models are presented. The extent to which they can foster collaboration and address the redesign challenges are then examined.

Challenges in Hospital-Physician Relationships

Hospitals and physicians are products of two very different institutionalized cultures, involving bureaucracy in the case of hospitals and professional autonomy in the case of physicians[8] (see Chapters Two, Five, and Eight). Bureaucracies' need for economies of scale, mass production, efficiency, conformity, and predictability do not match up well with physicians' needs for on-demand resources, flexibility, discretion in decision making, and individualized patient care. The differences are more than surface deep. They embrace the nature of employment, the basis of knowledge and view of evidence, the focus of attention, the time frame of action, and the nature of resources (see Table 3.1).

Although almost all health care professional and support staff working in hospitals are hospital employees, most physicians are not. Therefore, the set of legal rights and obligations set forth in the employment contract is missing. The basis of knowledge for the top management team and governing board for most hospitals comes largely from the behavioral, social, and managerial sciences, whereas that of physicians comes primarily from the biological and life sciences. Health care

TABLE 3.1   CULTURAL DIFFERENCES BETWEEN HOSPITAL EXECUTIVES AND PHYSICIANS

Attribute	Hospital Executives	Physicians
Relationship to the organization	Employed	Voluntary medical staff member
Primary basis of knowledge	Behavioral, managerial, and social sciences	Biological and life sciences
View of evidence	Experiential, "colloquial," observational, cost and benefit	Randomized clinical trial
Focus	All patients, the community	My patient
Time frame of action	Weeks or months, strategic plans, budget cycles	Short-run or immediate; the patient in front of me
View of resources	Always limited	Should be unlimited for my patient
Professional identity	Relatively weak	Strong
Overall gestalt	Physicians exist to help meet the overall goals of the hospital	Hospital exists to help me care for my patients and advance my professional career

Source: Authors' analysis.

executives largely draw on evidence in an eclectic fashion from multiple sources, much of it "colloquial,"[9] whereas physicians take as their starting point evidence that is drawn largely from randomized clinical trials and related approaches (even though this evidence may not be routinely applied in practice). The hospital management team is focused on *all* patients in the hospital, whereas physicians are focused mainly on their *individual* patients. The time frame in which hospital executives make decisions is usually the medium to long term and is characterized by strategic plans, budget cycles, and monthly reports. In contrast, the time frame in which physicians often must act is within minutes (for example, "What do I do with the patient in front of me?" or, "What do I do with the emergency case that just came in the door?"). Finally, hospital executives fully realize that all resources are limited, and the challenge is to deploy them in a way that will optimize their return in order to achieve the hospital's goals. Physicians, in contrast, are often aware that resources are limited, but believe that they should not deprive their own patients of resources.

The institutionalized cultural divide between hospitals and physicians can be summed up by noting that from the hospital's perspective, physicians exist to work with the hospital to achieve its goals. In contrast, from the physicians' perspective, the hospital exists to help the physicians meet their goals for their patients and to advance the physician's professional career.

These different institutional forces are also influenced by different market forces across the country. Most prominent among these are the degree of competition between and among physicians and hospitals, the various forms and amounts of payment and reimbursement available, and different regulatory and legal policies and practices (see Chapters Four and Six). In general, the greater the degree of market competition, payment pressures, and regulatory intensity, the greater the stress on the hospital-physician relationship and the division between the bureaucratic and the autonomy cultures. Thus, both market and institutional forces pose challenges to developing collaborative hospital-physician relationships.[10]

Given these points, it is helpful to consider the nature of the exchange relationship between hospitals and physicians on a continuum from transactional to relational. *Transactional* exchanges involve highly instrumental, arm's-length, market-based, contractual transactions between the parties involved. *Relational* exchanges involve a high degree of intrinsic agreement and commitment to a shared set of goals.[11] These exchanges usually occur when the parties involved are employed by the same organization, have an exclusive relationship, or have a high degree of intensive interaction with each other. Relational exchanges significantly lower the transaction costs of doing business and facilitate trust. The construct underlying the continuum is the degree of commitment to shared goals. More relational exchanges will result in a greater degree of hospital-physician integration and better working relationships. An important question is the extent to which transactional exchanges between hospitals and physicians can be designed in such a way as to also promote more effective working relationships.

The test of the relationship is the extent to which the six Institute of Medicine redesign challenges can be addressed. Table 3.2 shows how each of these might

TABLE 3.2   THE INSTITUTE OF MEDICINE'S REDESIGN CHALLENGES AND THE TRANSACTIONAL-RELATIONAL CONTINUUM

Redesign Challenges	Transactional ⟶ Relational	
Redesign care processes	Separation of office practices from hospital practices; ad hoc committee work on quality improvement processes	Protocols and pathways established for entire episode of care, embracing both inpatient and ambulatory care; disease management teams work seamlessly with primary care physicians and hospital staff
Effective use of information technology (IT) (electronic health records and the like)	Hospitals and physicians make independent decisions; work with independent vendors	Coordinated IT strategy established after redesigning patient care workflow; work with common vendor
Knowledge and skills management	Occurs largely in isolation and by chance; uses traditional clinical education programs	Uses IT capability to generate real-time data for knowledge and upgrading of skills; uses custom-designed, problem-focused learning
Develop effective teams	Separation between hospital teams and private practice teams; separate team development programs	Continuum of care–based team development; disease management team training includes inpatient, out-patient, and at-home care
Coordination of care across patient conditions, providers, and settings over time	Accomplished through integrating referral arrangements and contracts; little monitoring or feedback	Designed into one care plan across settings and providers; use of common electronic health records helps with flow of information and feedback
Performance and outcome measurement	Largely ad hoc, accreditation-oriented, separation of hospital indicators from ambulatory indicators	Integrative scorecard; set of indicators used for quality improvement and external reporting

Source: Authors' analysis.

be addressed under a transactional approach and under a relational approach. The subsequent discussion of the four different accountable care organization models will use the transactional-relational continuum in regard to developing collaborative relationships and addressing the redesign challenges.

Accountable Care Organizations (ACOs)

Most health care today is provided in silos of hospitals, physician practices, clinics, ambulatory surgery centers, nursing homes, home health agencies, and other sites. Each faces a different set of incentives and constraints. Each treats a part of the patient. Each works from a somewhat different base of patient information. This system is "designed" for suboptimization, as each part works to optimize its performance with little, if any, consideration for the other parts. This system is "designed" to produce errors, duplicate testing, and leave gaps in information and communication, resulting in a highly variable quality of care and high costs. These problems are exacerbated by the growing number of Americans with chronic illnesses, who frequently require care across multiple providers and settings.

What are needed are delivery models that bring these parts together to provide care that is better coordinated and integrated for the patient. The overarching template for such models is the *accountable care organization* (ACO)—also referred to as the *accountable care system* (ACS).[12] An ACO is an entity that is clinically and fiscally accountable for the entire continuum of care that a given population of patients may need. The ACOs have two primary responsibilities. The first responsibility is to continuously improve the value of the care delivered to patients. Value is defined as the quality, outcomes of care, and patient satisfaction divided by the cost of providing care.[13] The second responsibility is to provide data that document the value achieved for purposes of external accountability.

To accomplish these two major responsibilities, ACOs must do the following:

- Establish an administrative and governance structure that can provide leadership and accountability for the care that is provided
- Be able to measure costs, quality, and outcomes of care
- Be able to aggregate and report the data
- Have sufficient numbers of patients within targeted diagnostic categories to detect statistically significant and clinically relevant differences from desired benchmarks of performance
- Have the necessary infrastructure of clinical information technology and work process redesign capability to continuously improve care.

Current experience also suggests that ACOs need to be able to provide primary preventive care services, ensure twenty-four-hour coverage, coordinate the use of specialty care, and participate in care management and quality improvement activities.[14]

There are also desired attributes of patient-centered medical homes, which can serve as a key building block for ACOs.[15] ACOs meeting these criteria have the potential to bring together the different components of the health system to provide high-value care. Whether or not they can achieve this potential will depend, importantly, on whether they can successfully bridge the chasm that frequently exists between hospitals and physicians: the cultural divide between bureaucracy and professional autonomy and the different incentives promoting such division.

Four ACO Models

The ACO concept recognizes the importance of offering hospitals and physicians choice in how they work with each other. This is particularly important given the heterogeneity of local health care markets in the United States and the historical evolution of hospital and physician relationships across the country. Four different ACO models with the potential to provide more effective hospital-physician relationships are considered. Some involve integration and some are examples of alignment. The models are the *integrated delivery system* (IDS), sometimes called the *organized delivery system*; the *multispecialty group practice* (MSGP); the *physician hospital organization* (PHO); and the *independent practice association* (IPA) and its variations.

The IDSs and MSGPs that work exclusively with a single health system are, by definition, integrated ACO models. The remaining two—PHOs and IPAs—are alignment models, designed to bring physicians and hospitals closer together in varying degrees (more so for the PHO than the IPA). In regard to these two models, it is important to note that nearly 70 percent of the care provided to Medicare beneficiaries is delivered by physicians within local hospital-physician networks (also called *natural referral networks*), and much of the additional care is delivered by an obvious referral source.[16] This suggests that the major barriers to integration or alignment lie in the inherent challenges of establishing the formal organizational relationships needed to accept accountability for cost and quality, and in the alignment of financial and professional incentives to accomplish key tasks to achieve more cost-effective care.

The IDS

Integrated delivery systems can be defined as administrative entities that bring together a set of organizations that provide a coordinated continuum of services to a defined population and are willing to be held clinically and fiscally accountable for the outcomes and health status of the population served.[17] This is essentially the same as the definition for an ACO, except that it recognizes that multiple organizations may need to be brought together into a system. Most IDSs emerged from multihospital systems, which added physicians, ambulatory surgery centers, home health agencies, nursing homes, and related components over time. Some IDSs, such as Kaiser Permanente, Group Health Cooperative of Puget Sound, and the Veterans Health Administration own all of the component hospitals and health plans with an employed physician staff or exclusive relationship with physician group practices. Thus they are in the best position to reduce the transaction costs and establish relational properties between hospitals and physicians. Others are hybrid models of hospitals and clinics, with or without owned insurance plans. Examples include the Cleveland Clinic, the Geisinger Health System, InterMountain Health Care, Henry Ford Health System, Sharp HealthCare, and Sutter Health. IDSs, by their very nature, are prime candidates to serve as ACOs in that most possess the administrative and governance structure, data collection analysis and reporting capacity, clinical information technology and work process redesign capabilities, and have a significant volume of patients—all necessary criteria for a functioning ACO.

There is a growing but not yet definitive body of literature on the performance of IDSs in regard to quality and cost.[18] Overall, it suggests that IDSs provide as good or better quality of care at the same or lower cost than the more loosely organized, largely fee-for-service systems of care. Some of this evidence is limited to studies of very highly integrated systems such as Kaiser Permanente or the Veterans Health Administration,[19] but there is also evidence of superior performance by other IDSs.[20] Although more definitive research is needed, an important reason for the better performance appears to be the ability of IDSs to provide more coordinated, team-based care to patients with chronic illness, supported by a high degree of electronic health record functionality.

The MSGP

There are at least 210 multispecialty group practices of fifty or more physicians in the United States.[21] These groups have long been known for their ability to have physicians from multiple specialties work together to care for their patients. This is increasingly important given the growing prevalence of chronic illness, frequently requiring multiple providers. MSGPs may also have access to capital, capable leaders, and a strong group culture that facilitates adapting to changes. Because they include multiple specialties, they can provide most care that patients need within the group, facilitate patient referral, improve care coordination, and make the group more capable of overseeing all the costs of the patient's care. This is particularly true for those MSGPs that are closely aligned with hospitals or that have their own hospitals, such as the Mayo Clinic and Virginia Mason Medical Center. These arrangements reduce transaction costs, increase the degree to which goals are shared, and build trust.

Existing evidence suggests that large MSGPs have more clinical information technology, use more organized processes to improve care, are more likely to participate in quality improvement activities, and are more likely to score well on process measures of quality than are less organized or integrated physicians.[22] There is also evidence that they perform more recommended prevention services.[23] Larger groups also meet more criteria for serving as a patient-centered medical home,[24] including having more clinical information technology.[25] But a study of Massachusetts practices found no relationship between group size and higher performance scores on Healthcare Effectiveness Data and Information Set (HEDIS) measures.[26] Research is needed to compare larger and smaller practices on a broader set of quality and outcomes of care.

The PHO

The physician hospital organization is an entity that brings together physicians and hospitals in a formal relationship that can both provide and contract with health plans for hospital and physician services. As such, PHOs have potential for achieving some degree of shared goal commitment and lie in the middle of the transactional-relational continuum. Early PHOs emerged in response to the Medicare Prospective Payment System (see Chapter Four) as a means to provide incentives for physicians to reduce inpatient costs. Subsequent growth was largely tied to the expansion of managed care and the opportunities offered to both physicians and hospitals under capitated payment models. Many PHOs, however, lacked the ability to provide more cost-effective care. As patients and providers alike rebelled against the restrictions of tightly managed care and as capitated payment became less prevalent, PHOs began to decline. However, there remain at least several hundred PHOs today, ranging from a single hospital that employs some or all of its specialist and primary care physicians to multihospital systems, such as Advocate Health System in Chicago, which establish contractual relationships with physicians in office practices.

The potential of the PHO as a vehicle for achieving accountability for cost and quality across the care continuum lies in several elements. As discussed earlier, most physicians already practice within natural referral networks around one hospital. Recent studies have found that hospitals are increasingly employing not only primary care physicians but also specialist physicians, as voluntary participation in hospital-based activities on the part of medical staff physicians declines.[27] Hospitals have an organizational infrastructure and resources that could be used to support clinical integration across inpatient and outpatient sites of care. Without some source of support, small physician office practices will be hard-pressed to adopt the electronic health records, care management systems, and other infrastructure required to improve both the quality and efficiency of care. Nonetheless, at this point in time, there is no systematic evidence on the cost or quality performance of PHOs.

The IPA

Many independent practice associations continue to serve primarily as vehicles for contracting with health plans. As such, they lie closer to the transactional end of the continuum than the relational, making it more difficult to achieve alignment between hospitals and physicians. Some, however, bring together individual, often small, physician practices into a coordinated virtual network of physicians that can provide more cost-effective patient care, rather than merely providing support services for insurance plan contracting. Examples include Hill Physicians Group in Northern California, Health Partners in Los Angeles (also an MSGP), and Monarch in Southern California—all functioning under California's delegated model of capitation for commercial HMO enrollees. These IPAs provide support to implement electronic health records, chronic care management processes, quality improvement goals, and related infrastructure. Given common payment incentives, these *practice redesign* IPAs have greater potential for achieving integration with hospitals than do the historical *contracting* IPAs.

Virtual IPAs could be particularly attractive to smaller practices and those in rural areas that otherwise lack the infrastructure and resources to create a true IPA and qualify as an ACO on their own. Examples of virtual IPAs include the North Carolina Community Consortium, which largely serves Medicaid patients,[28] the Grand Junction Colorado Physician Network,[29] the North Dakota Physician Network, and Humboldt County California Physician Network. When practices come together into a virtual network of practices, they create economies of scale and capabilities in data collection, analysis, and reporting; aggregate a sufficient number of patients to qualify for incentive payments; and provide technical assistance for implementing electronic health records and supporting work process redesign. These arrangements also provide an alternative to those physicians who fear large formal bureaucratic organizations as represented by IDSs, PHOs, or even MSGPs.[30] Given that over 30 percent of physicians practice in groups of nine doctors or fewer, IPAs and virtual IPA arrangements may have the greatest potential for growth.

IPAs have less electronic health record functionality than multispecialty medical groups and are less likely to participate in quality improvement programs, but there is no difference in their use of recommended care management processes.[31] There is relatively little systematic evidence on the actual cost or quality performance of IPAs and related arrangements.

Promoting Hospital-Physician Collaboration

The four models—IDSs, MSGPs, PHOs, and IPAs—have varying potential for promoting greater collaboration between hospitals and physicians. Overall, the IDS and exclusive MSGP models have the greatest potential for promoting the type of physician-hospital collaboration likely to be required by new payment incentives (see Chapter Four).

The key to collaboration is the ability of hospitals and physicians to commit to shared goals and to develop the capabilities to realize those goals. This involves establishing trust. As shown in the upper-left-hand cell in Figure 3.2, a healthy relationship with a high degree of collaboration exists where physicians have a high level of trust in the organization *and* a high level of perceived degree of control over their work and involvement in decision making. The upper-right-hand cell depicts the situation of hospital dominance where physician trust in the organization is high but physicians' perceived control is low. This can be a viable but highly fragile relationship. In general, one would expect a relatively low degree of collaboration in these relationships. The lower-left-hand cell depicts the situation of physician dominance, in which physicians perceive a high degree of

FIGURE 3.2   PHYSICIAN-ORGANIZATION RELATIONSHIPS

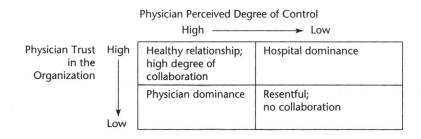

Source: Adapted from S. M. Shortell, R. R. Gillies, D. A. Anderson, K. Erickson, and others, *Remaking Health Care in America: Building Organized Delivery Systems, 2nd ed.* (San Francisco: Jossey-Bass, 2000), p. 78.

control but have little trust in the organization. Physicians will attempt to exert their dominance at the expense of larger hospital or systemwide goals. Thus, one can expect relatively low levels of collaboration in these situations as well. In the lower-right-hand cell, physicians neither trust the organization nor perceive any significant degree of control, resulting in the absence of collaboration and most likely a high degree of conflict and resentment on the part of both parties.

A number of factors have been identified to successfully overcome such conflicts. As shown in Figure 3.3, these include the foundational properties of leadership and empowerment (also see Chapter Eight), governance and management (also see Chapter Seven) and capital resources. These, in turn, give rise to five robust properties that are likely to promote effective collaborative relationships regardless of any specific structural models or changes in the external environment. These include shared and aligned financial incentives, implementation of evidence-based care management practices, investment in clinical information technology, use

FIGURE 3.3   KEY FACTORS FOR ACHIEVING HOSPITAL-PHYSICIAN INTEGRATION

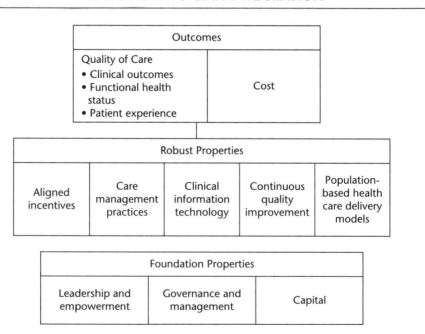

Source: Adapted from S. M. Shortell, R. R. Gillies, D. A. Anderson, K. Erickson, and others, *Remaking Health Care in America: Building Organized Delivery Systems, 2nd ed.* (San Francisco: Jossey-Bass, 2000), p. 92.

of continuous quality improvement methods, and adoption of population-based health delivery models.[32] These are the building-block processes of hospital-physician integration to produce improved quality and outcomes of care and improve patient experience at lower cost.

IDSs have great potential for developing strong collaborative relationships between hospitals and physicians. This is primarily due to their relational arrangements with their physicians through direct employment or exclusive contractual relationships. Many IDSs also have transactional relationships with other physicians practicing in the community who serve as members of the IDS's voluntary medical staff. In this case, most IDSs use their employed MSGP to influence the behavior of the more loosely coupled physicians. This is done through the selection of referral partners and through exerting soft forms of persuasion to use IDS guidelines, protocols, information systems, and quality improvement processes. Many IDSs also provide direct practice support services to these loosely coupled physicians to encourage greater alignment of interest.

Although IDSs have great potential for promoting a high degree of collaboration, it is important to recognize that there is considerable heterogeneity across IDSs. For example, in a comparative study of eleven IDSs, clinical and system leaders rated the degree of physician-system integration as only 2.6 on a scale in which 1 represented a low degree of integration and 5 represented a high degree of integration. One respondent noted: "What doctor wants to think of his or her goal as fitting into a system?"[33] Major barriers in addition to distrust of large organizations included conflict between primary care physicians and specialists over practice styles, referral relationships, payment, and resources; lack of physician leadership; and weak or nonexistent clinical information systems.

Thus, integrated delivery systems vary in the extent to which they possess the foundational and robust properties outlined in Figure 3.3. However, most have the capital to invest in the robust properties and are of sufficient size to develop population-based delivery models. But IDSs are also expensive to develop and challenging to create through mergers and acquisitions. Further, it takes time to build a culture of trust among the parties involved. As a result, it is unlikely that the number of IDSs will grow significantly in the future, but a sufficient number currently exists across the country to serve as the backbone for ACO formation.

The extent to which MSGPs can promote greater hospital-physician collaboration will depend, as suggested by Figure 3.2, on the relative degree of trust and perceived control that the MSGP has relative to its associated hospital. Physicians' perceptions of trust and control will depend on the percentage of admissions to the hospital and the extent to which the MSGP physicians play important leadership roles in the hospital. This, in turn, will depend on the extent to which the MSGP possesses the foundational and robust properties outlined in Figure 3.3. Many but not all multispecialty groups have the capital, the governance and management structure, the culture, and the leadership to develop robust properties, particularly in regard to implementing care management processes, clinical information technology, and continuous quality improvement processes.

It is also important to note the extent to which multispecialty medical groups that are not part of an IDS possess various options in functioning as an ACO. For example, they could join and create a PHO with one or more hospitals and most likely other physicians as well. Second, they could choose to function as an independent ACO on their own. Third, they could join with other physicians to form a mixed-model MSGP–virtual physician organization. In any of these options, it will be difficult for the group to improve the overall quality and reduce the overall cost of care without cooperation from the hospitals to which patients are admitted. Therefore, if the second or third options were chosen and the relevant hospital(s) were not part of the ACO, the physicians would need enough leverage to induce hospital cooperation by the implicit and explicit threat of moving admissions to competing hospitals. This type of adversarial relationship could be avoided, however, by including the hospital in shared savings or bonuses received by the ACO. Further, the hospitals will have additional incentives to cooperate if they are rewarded through pay-for-performance for lowering the rate of hospital readmissions and related indicators.

PHOs have the potential for bridging the chasm between hospitals and physicians, but this is highly dependent on the quality of leadership that exists from both parties, and on the relative balance of power. Most hospital organizations have little experience managing physician practices, and the relationship between hospital leadership and physicians has often been difficult. Physicians, particularly those in primary care, may fear losing power within organizations that may be dominated by hospitals, especially as decisions are made about how to distribute shared savings or other financial incentives. Finally, data from regional studies suggests that a large fraction of the potential waste in the current delivery system is related to the unnecessary use of the hospital as a site of care.[34] PHOs dominated by powerful hospitals may be unwilling to consider serious strategies for improving efficiency that result in lower inpatient revenues.

Of the four ACO models, the IPAs face the greatest challenge in developing the foundation of robust properties to promote hospital-physician collaboration. Most small physician practices throughout the United States lack the capital to invest in the robust properties and also vary greatly in the extent to which physicians have the time, interest, or ability to play the necessary leadership roles, develop the cultural norms and values, and forge the necessary governance and management structures.

A common problem in physician-hospital relationships is the inability of the physicians to speak with a common voice in their discussions with hospitals. IPAs can provide this voice to the extent there is strong administrative and governance leadership that can speak on behalf of its members. This can help position the IPA in the upper-left-hand cell in Figure 3.2, promoting a high degree of trust between physicians and the hospital, and with physicians perceiving a high degree of influence. New payment reforms and public reporting requirements will create incentives for IPA physicians and hospitals to work together more closely. The IPA will provide a platform for these hospitals and physicians to respond to the incentives.

Formation of the IPA could thus move the physician-hospital relationship from being primarily transactional to more relational. This will be reflected in the development of agreed-upon treatment guidelines, protocols for prevalent conditions, more standardized and compatible systems for electronic health record information transfer, and the development of shared performance reporting systems. IPAs, or virtual IPAs, are likely to be particularly attractive in rural areas where there often exists a close relationship with the local hospital (see Chapter Eleven). In these cases, the ACO is the IPA with its local hospital, whether or not a formal PHO is created. In suburban and urban communities, IPAs may include multiple hospitals as part of the ACO. In these situations, as previously noted, the ability of the IPA to induce desired hospital behavior will depend on both the volume of patients that can be directed to the various hospitals and the quality of the administrative and governance leadership of the IPA to speak with authority and credibility on behalf of its physicians. Overall, creating more grouplike IPAs will depend on the development of strong payment incentives, public reporting requirements, technical assistance, and resources. Without such incentives and support, relatively few small physician practices or the current loosely coupled IPAs will have the motivation to transform themselves into robust IPAs.

Addressing the Redesign Imperatives

The IDS is well positioned to address each of the six Institute of Medicine redesign challenges shown in Table 3.2. This is primarily because IDSs embrace the entire continuum of care and have the greatest number of relational properties among the component parts. By employing at least a major portion of their physicians, IDSs have the potential to integrate physician goals with those of the hospital. The development of shared goals, values, and norms permits greater collaboration and the development of more cost-effective approaches for patient treatment; teamwork to coordinate care across settings; and sharing of knowledge and best practices. The IDSs have the capital, the size, and the technical expertise to implement electronic health records and to produce relevant performance data on quality and cost for both external reporting and internal continuous quality improvement. Even where physicians are not employed, IDSs have the resources and infrastructure to encourage closer alignment between the hospital and the physicians, assuming that changes in public policy regarding payment and legal and regulatory reforms are implemented (see Chapters Four and Six).

MSGPs must rely heavily on the governance and management leadership of the group and its relationships to involved hospitals to address the redesign challenges. The leadership of the group will need to work with the leadership of the hospital, for example, in ensuring that patients and family members understand discharge instructions, know the warning signs of their illness, have an adequate supply of medications and know how to use them, and have a follow-up appointment with the appropriate physician. The practice would need to work with the hospital to ensure that the patient's physicians are informed when the patient is discharged and that they receive discharge summaries and relevant information within twenty-four hours of discharge. The multispecialty physician practices could track patients after discharge and contact them immediately if they miss a follow-up appointment. Physicians could also use a variety of care management processes—for example, tracking chronically ill patients with registries, teaching patients self-management skills, using nurse care managers for patients with severe chronic illness, providing patients with electronic access to their medical records and ready e-mail or phone access to staff and physicians.

Although the processes to improve care and reduce readmissions could be most easily implemented in an IDS with command and control authority, they could also be implemented in MSGPs, depending on the incentives. For example, if Medicare payments to hospitals are reduced for readmissions, hospitals would have a strong incentive to invest in these processes, but physicians would not. In this case, hospitals that employ the physicians would be able to implement the processes for these physicians. But physicians not employed by the hospital would have no financial incentives to cooperate with the hospital to reduce readmissions. However, if they were part of an MSGP ACO, even if not included in the hospital, the physicians would have an incentive to help the hospital reduce readmissions because this would be important to the ACO's effort to control the total cost to its patients. An ongoing challenge, however, involves the extent to which the electronic records used by hospitals are compatible and interoperable with the system used by the MSGP. Successfully dealing with this issue will greatly influence the ability of the multispecialty group ACO model to address the related redesign challenges as well.

PHOs may have a slight advantage over freestanding MSGPs in addressing the redesign challenges involved in the physician-hospital relationship. This is because there is a formal governance and administrative structure that involves both the hospital and the physicians. Thus, it should be somewhat easier for the PHO to work on the redesign challenges. In particular, there would be forums in place to design interventions to improve care processes, develop interdisciplinary teams to coordinate care across settings, and to do performance measurement and continuous quality improvement. But a number of challenges would still remain. In particular, although an IDS can purchase and deploy a single electronic health record, a hospital with many practices making up the PHO is unlikely to do so. This results in the challenges of interoperability and the associated technical and political issues previously noted.

As noted, the new IPAs are organizations of physician practices linked together in a partnership to improve quality and contain cost under new performance measurement and public reporting incentives and requirements. IPAs, of course, will be much more loosely organized than IDSs but will also be less tightly structured than MSGPs and PHOs. Thus, they will need more help to redesign care, implement electronic health records, develop knowledge and skill management systems, use teams, coordinate care across settings over time, and measure performance. Possible sources for such assistance include the local hospital, local foundations, quality improvement organizations under the Centers for Medicare and Medicaid Services (CMS), or the development of a new CMS Center for Innovations in Healthcare Delivery. Still another approach would be to provide incentives that pair existing exemplary IDSs and MSGPs to provide assistance, a concept called *organizational mentoring*, or *twinning*. Particularly important will be the ability of the IPAs to implement interoperable electronic health records, aggregate performance data, make use of quality improvement processes, and share and identify best practices across the network. Innovations, such as the development of teams of nurses, pharmacists, and social workers that serve multiple cross-site practices, will also be needed. Individual practices cannot accomplish these activities alone. But the experiences of North Carolina; Grand Junction, Colorado; North Dakota; and Humboldt County, California provide examples of what can be accomplished with strong leadership.

A Supporting Framework for Developing ACOs

As shown in Figure 3.4, the following will be needed to promote ACOs across the country: financial incentives, regulatory flexibility, and the development of internal capabilities and transparent accountability generated by performance measurement

FIGURE 3.4   SUPPORTIVE FRAMEWORK FOR CREATING ACCOUNTABLE CARE ORGANIZATIONS (ACOS)

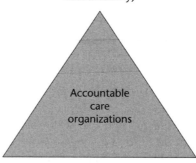

Transparent accountability
(performance measurement and public
accountability)

Accountable
care
organizations

Financial incentives and regulatory
flexibility (for example, bundled
payments, shared savings)

Internal capabilities (for
example, electronic health
records, governance and
administrative leadership)

Source: Authors' analysis.

and public reporting. Key to all three is the patient choice of an ACO or assignment to one based on current and past utilization experience. Research suggests that over 80 percent of patients continue to see physicians affiliated with the same ACO, so such assignment is feasible.[35]

Payment Reform and Regulatory Flexibility

ACOs could be paid a number of different ways (also see Chapter Four). For example, spending targets for Medicare patients based on the most recent three years of utilization and cost data,[36] bundled payments for selected conditions and procedures (for example, coronary artery bypass grafts and total hip or total knee replacements), and bonus payments to physicians willing to assume care coordination responsibility for all of a patient's care while meeting predetermined quality criteria.

Medicare spending targets would include an allowance for spending growth and would be adjusted for differences in area wage rates. Provided quality targets were met (for example, preventable mortality, ambulatory care sensitive hospital admissions, preventable readmissions, patient satisfaction, HEDIS process measures, and so on), the ACO would receive a bonus if it stayed within its spending target. This would create aligned financial incentives for all members of the ACO—for example, for participating physicians, hospitals, home health agencies, and nursing homes. Risk-adjusted bundled payments (in other words, single payment for both the hospital and physician for selected conditions) could be incorporated within the spending target as an additional incentive. This would provide an opportunity for some ACOs to receive additional revenues even if they did not meet their overall spending target. The same could apply for those who might receive additional care coordination payments. To encourage a strong foundation of primary care, additional payments could be made to ACOs to establish patient-centered medical homes.[37]

Payment might also vary by level of ACO eligibility. A balance must be struck between encouraging physicians and hospitals to join ACOs to be eligible for rewards and the need for sufficiently stringent standards to induce desired behavior. Basic (or level 1) eligibility criteria for being paid as an ACO might include the following:

- Having a legal entity with a designated governance and leadership-management team in place
- Encompassing a specific minimum number of practices, patient-centered medical homes, a hospital, and specialists to meet the needs of the designated population served
- Having a sufficient volume of patients (for example, a minimum of 15,000) to be able to report cost and quality data
- Having basic lab and medication data on all patients.

Level 2 ACOs might add evidence of using disease registries, guidelines, and patient reminder systems and having increased electronic health record functionality. Level 3 might add

- Making full use of care management processes, including patient self-management programs
- Using nurse case managers
- Having pharmacist-led medication teams
- Participating in ongoing quality improvement activities
- Having fully functional, interoperable electronic health records

These are intended only as examples, with a fine line to be drawn between being overly prescriptive on the one hand and setting the bar too low on the other hand. Payment and incentive rewards would vary by level, with level 3

ACOs being eligible for the greatest gains but also facing the greatest risk, such as under global capitation. Level 1 would receive the least rewards, and level 2 would be eligible for intermediate rewards—again consistent with the degree of risk assumed. Establishing levels of eligibility will allow smaller practices to qualify at the base level, while giving them incentives to develop their capabilities to advance to higher levels over time. One example of this approach is the Pittsburgh Regional Health Initiative, which has established an accountable care network of 278 small practices that likely would qualify as level 1 or 2 ACOs, a situation most likely to be the case for many more loosely organized IPAs and smaller practices across the country.[38]

The use of spending targets or incentives that might result in the sharing of savings between hospitals and physicians is also subject to current legal restrictions on gainsharing (see Chapter Six). Further, as hospitals and physician practices aggregate in size, they are subject to potential antitrust concerns. Thus, attention also needs to be paid to mitigating the legal and regulatory barriers to encourage greater hospital and physician collaboration and formation of ACOs.

Capabilities and Accountability

Among the internal capabilities necessary for the formation of ACOs, the most important are the establishment of the governance and administrative leadership of the organization, the adoption and implementation of electronic health records, and development of a strong primary care base. Joint hospital and physician leadership is needed to establish the governance-administrative structure for the ACO that can make decisions, provide evidence-based medicine and management, and hold people accountable for the cost and quality of care. This will be a particular challenge for the IPA and virtual models due to the likely small size of many physician practices in this model.

Implementation of electronic health records is needed to perform the care coordination, quality improvement, performance measurement, and public reporting functions. Some ACOs, particularly those composed of small practices, will need technical assistance from Medicare Quality Improvement Organizations (or the other sources previously noted) to implement electronic health records with the functionality required to succeed as an ACO.

In addition, the most successful ACOs are likely to be those that develop a strong primary care base built on the patient-centered medical home model. A new primary care extension cooperative service, modeled after the U.S. Department of Agriculture's Cooperative Extension System, could be developed to assist in the development of patient-centered medical homes.[39] The governance and administrative leadership of the ACO will need to assure an appropriate balance of influence among primary care physicians and clinicians, specialists and hospitals in order to maximize the most cost-effective provision of care across various settings and providers.

Finally, in order to receive payment as well as to foster learning, ACOs must both produce and have access to performance data and publicly reported data on quality and cost. The opportunity to benchmark performance locally, regionally, and nationally provides not only the basis for payment but also incentives for improvement and feedback on what is working.

Conclusion

With the supportive framework described earlier, ACOs have the potential to eliminate some of the fragmentation inherent in the U.S. health care delivery system. The major appeal is the ability to *fix accountability* for both the quality and cost of care across the patient experience and over time. Medicare, as the largest payer, can take the lead in stimulating the development of ACOs, but it is likely that private insurers will need to follow to create sufficient alignment of the financial incentives for the majority, if not all, of the ACO's patients.

Early evidence from the Physician Group Practice Demonstration suggests that these ACO-like organizations are providing significantly higher quality of care, although not yet resulting in significant cost savings.[40] Given the entrenched behavior on the part of both hospitals and physicians in response to old incentives, it is unlikely that significant cost savings or breakthrough improvements in quality will occur quickly. Rather than being a discouragement, this is a strong argument that public policy needs to support the immediate development of ACOs across the country to provide a foundation for future cost-effective delivery. The failure to do so will result in a delivery system that will become even more dysfunctional and overwhelmed, frustrating the efforts of hospitals and physicians (and other providers) alike.

Notes

1. J. Wennberg, and A. Gittelsohn, "Small Area Variation in Health Care Delivery," *Science* 182, no. 117 (1973), 1102–1108; J. Wennberg, E. Fisher, and J. Skinner, "Geography and the Debate over Medicare Reform," *Health Affairs* Web exclusive (February 13, 2002), w96–w114, http://content.healthaffairs.org/cgi/reprint/hlthaff.w2.96v1; E. Fisher, J. Wennberg, T. Stukel, and D. Gottleib, "Variations in the Longitudinal Efficiency of Academic Medical Centers," *Health Affairs* Web exclusive (October 7, 2004), VAR-19-32, http://content.healthaffairs.org/cgi/reprint/hlthaff.var.19v1; L. Baker, E. Fisher, and

J. Wennberg, "Variations in Hospital Resources Use for Medicare and Privately Insured Populations in California,"*Health Affairs* 27, no. 2 (2008): 123–34.

2. J. Wennberg and others, "Geography and the Debate over Medicare Reform"; Fisher and others, "Variations in the Longitudinal Efficiency of Academic Medical Centers"; E. Fisher, J. Wennberg, T. Stukel, D. Gottleib, and others, "The Implications of Regional Variations in Medicare Spending. Part 1: The Content, Quality, and Accessibility of Care,"*Annals of Internal Medicine* 138, no. 4 (2003), 273–87.

3. Fisher and others, "Variations in the Longitudinal Efficiency of Academic Medical Centers.

4. J. Wennberg, E. Fisher, T. Stukel, J. Skinner, and others, "Use of Hospitals, Physician Visits, and Hospice Care During Last Six Months of Life Among Cohorts Loyal to Highly Respected Hospitals in the United States."*British Medical Journal* 328 (2004): 607–10.

5. Fisher and others, "Variations in the Longitudinal Efficiency of Academic Medical Centers"; Fisher and others, "The Implications of Regional Variations in Medicare Spending." Part 1; B. Sirovich, P. Gallagher, J. Wennberg, and E. Fisher, "Discretionary Decision Making by Primary Care Physicians and the Cost of U.S. Health Care," *Health Affairs* 27, no. 3 (2008): 813–23; B. Sirovich, D. Gottleib, H. Welch, and E. Fisher, "Regional Variations in Health Care Intensity and Physician Perceptions of Quality of Care,"*Annals of Internal Medicine* 144, no. 9 (2006): 641–49; J. Skinner, D. Staiger, and E. Fisher, "Is Technological Change in Medicine Always Worth It? The Case of Acute Myocardial Infarction," *Health Affairs* 25, no. 2 (2006): 34–47; J. Wennberg, K. Bronner, J. Skinner, E. Fisher, and others, "Inpatient Care and Patients' Ratings of Their Hospital Experiences,"*Health Affairs* 28, no. 1 (2009): 103–12.

6. Institute of Medicine, *Crossing the Quality Chasm: A New Health System for the 21st Century* (Washington, D.C.: National Academies Press, 2001); Institute of Medicine, *Performance Measurement: Accelerating Improvement* (Washington, D.C.: National Academies Press, 2006); M. O'Kane, J. Corrigan, S. Foote, S. Tunis, and others, "Crossroads in Quality,"*Health Affairs* 27, no. 3 (2008): 749–58.

7. E. Fisher, M. McClellan, J. Bertko, S. Lieberman, and others, "Fostering Accountable Health Care: Moving Forward in Medicare,"*Health Affairs* 28, no. 2, (2009): 219–31; S. M. Shortell and L. P. Casalino, "Health Care Reform Requires Accountable Care Systems," *JAMA* 300, no. 1 (2008): 95–97; E. Fisher, "Building a Medical Neighborhood for the Medical Home,"*New England Journal of Medicine* 359, no. 12 (2008): 1202–05.

8. E. Freidson, *Profession of Medicine: A Study of the Sociology of Applied Knowledge* (New York: Dodd, Mead, 1970); E. Freidson, "The Changing Nature of Professional Control,"*Annual Review of Sociology* 10 (1984): 1–20; P. M. Starr, *The Social Transformation of American Medicine* (New York: Basic Books, 1982); T. G. Rundall, S. M. Shortell, and J. A. Alexander, "A Theory of Physician-Hospital Integration: Contending Institutional and Market Logics in the Health Care Field," *Journal of Health and Social Behavior* 45 (2004): S102–S117.

9. T. Rundall, P. Martelli, R. McCurdy, L. Arroyo, and others, "Using Research Evidence When Making Decisions: Views of Health Services Managers and Policy Makers," in *Evidence-Based Management in Health Care*, ed. A. Kovner, D. Aguila, and D. Fine (Chicago: Health Administration Press, 2009).

10. Rundall and others, "A Theory of Physician-Hospital Integration"; W. Scott, M. Ruef, P. Mendel, and L. Caronna, *Institutionalized Change and Healthcare Organizations: From Professional Dominance to Managed Care* (Chicago: University of Chicago Press, 2000); J. Alexander, and T. O'Aumo, "Alternative Perspectives on Institutional and Market Relationships in the U.S. Health Sector," in *Advances in Health Care Organization Theory*, ed. S. Mick and

M. E. Wyttenbach, 2nd ed. (San Francisco: Jossey-Bass, 2003) 45–77; L. Burns and R. Muller, "Hospital-Physician Collaboration: Landscape of Economics Integration and Impact on Clinical Integration," *Milbank Quarterly* 86, no. 3 (2008): 375–434.

11. D. Rousseau, *Psychological Contracts in Organizations: Understanding Written and Unwritten Agreements* (Thousand Oaks, CA: Sage, 1995).

12. Fisher and others, "Fostering Accountable Health Care"; Shortell and Casalino, "Health Care Reform Requires Accountable Care Systems"; Medicare Payment Advisory Commission, "Accountable Care Organizations," in *Report to Congress: Improving Incentives to the Medicare Program* (Washington, D.C.: Medicare Payment Advisory Commission, 2009) 39–60, http://www.medpac.gov/chapters/June09_Ch01.pdf (accessed June 25, 2009).

13. National Quality Forum, *Measurement Framework: Evaluating Efficiency Across Patient-Focused Episodes of Care* (Washington, D.C.: National Quality Forum, 2009).

14. D. McCarthy and K. Mueller, *Community Care of North Carolina: Building Community Systems of Care Through State and Local Partnerships* (New York: The Commonwealth Fund, 2009), 1–13.

15. D. Rittenhouse, L. Casalino, R. Gillies, S. Shortell, and others, "Measuring the Medical Home Infrastructure in Large Medical Groups," *Health Affairs* 27, no. 5 (2008): 1246–58; D. R. Rittenhouse and S. M. Shortell, "The Patient-Centered Medical Home: Can It Stand the Test of Healthcare Reform?" *JAMA* 301, no. 19 (2009): 2038–40.

16. J. Bynum, E. Bernald-Delgado, D. Gottlieb, and E. Fisher, "Assigning Ambulatory Patients and Their Physicians to Hospitals: A Method for Obtaining Population-Based Provider Performance Measures," *Health Services Research* 41, no. 1, pt. 1 (2007): 45–62.

17. S. M. Shortell, R. R. Gillies, D. A. Anderson, K. Erickson, and others, *Remaking Health Care in America: Building Organized Delivery Systems* (San Francisco: Jossey-Bass, 1996).

18. L. P. Casalino, "Which Type of Medical Group Provides Higher Quality Care?" *Annals of Internal Medicine* 145 (2006): 860–61; L. Tollen, *Physician Organization in Relation to Quality and Efficiency of Care: A Synthesis of Recent Literature* (New York: The Commonwealth Fund, 2008).

19. R. Feachem, N. Sekhri, and K. White, "Getting More for Their Dollar: A Comparison of the NHS with California's Kaiser Permanente," *British Medical Journal* 324 (2002): 135–43; C. Ham, N. York, S. Sutch, and R. Shaw, "Hospital Bed Utilisation in the NHS, Kaiser Permanente, and the US Medicare Programme: Analysis of Routine Data," *British Medical Journal* 327 (2003): 1257; A. Jha, J. Perlin, K. Kizer, and R. Dudley, "Effect of the Transformation of the Veterans Affairs Health Care System on the Quality of Care," *New England Journal of Medicine* 348, no. 22 (2003): 2218–27; S. Asch, E. McGlynn, M. Hogan, R. Hayward, and others, "Comparison of Quality of Care for Patients in the Veterans Health Administration and Patients in a National Sample," *Annals of Internal Medicine* 141, no. 12 (2004): 938–45; E. Kerr, R. Gerzoff, N. Krein, J. Selby, and others, "Diabetes Care Quality in the Veterans Affairs Health Care System and Commercial Managed Care: The Triad Study," *Annals of Internal Medicine* 141, no. 4 (2004): 272–81.

20. R. Gillies, K. Chenok, S. Shortell, G. Pawlson, and others, "The Impact of Health Plan Delivery System Organization on Clinical Quality and Patient Satisfaction," *Health Services Research* 41, no. 4, pt. 1 (2006), 1181–99; S. M. Shortell and J. Schmittdiel, "Prepaid Groups and Organized Delivery Systems: Promise, Performance, and Potential," in *Toward a 21st Century Health System*, ed. A. Enthoven and L. Tollen, 1–21 (San Francisco: Jossey-Bass, 2004).

21. *National Study of Physician Organizations II* (Berkeley: School of Public Health, University of California, 2007).

22. Tollen, *Physician Organization in Relation to Quality and Efficiency of Care*; A. Mehrotra, A. Epstein, and M. Rosenthal, "Do Integrated Medical Groups Provide Higher-Quality Medical Care Than IPAs?"*Annals of Internal Medicine* 145, no. 11 (2006): 826–33; L. Casalino, R. R. Gillies, S. M. Shortell, J. A. Schmittdiel, and others, "External Incentives, Information Technology, and Organized Processes to Improve Health Care Quality for Patients with Chronic Diseases," *JAMA* 289, no. 4 (2003): 434–41.

23. J. Schmittdiel, S. McMenamin, H. Halpin, R. Gillies, and others, "The Use of Patient and Physician Reminders for Preventive Services: Results from the National Study of Physician Organizations,"*Preventive Medicine* 39, no. 5 (2004): 1000–06; S. McMenamin, J. Schmittdiel, H. Halpin, R. Gillies, and others, "Health Promotion in Physician Organizations: Results from a National Survey,"*American Journal of Preventive Medicine* 26 (2004): 259–64; H. Pham, D. Schrag, J. Hargraves, and P. Back, "Delivery of Preventive Services to Older Adults by Primary Care Physicians," *JAMA* 294, no. 4 (2005): 473–81.

24. Rittenhouse and others, "Measuring the Medical Home Infrastructure in Large Medical Groups."

25. D. Rittenhouse and J. Robinson, "Improving Quality in Medicaid: The Use of Care Management Processes for Chronic Illness and Preventive Care,"*Medical Care* 44, no. 1 (2006): 47–54; J. Robinson, L. Casalino, R. Gillies, D. Rittenhouse, and others, "Financial Incentives, Quality Improvement Programs, and the Adoption of Clinical Information Technology," *Medical Care* 47, no. 4 (2009): 411–17.

26. M. Friedberg, K. Coltin, S. Pearon, K. Kleinman, and others, "Does Affiliation of Physician Groups with One Another Produce Higher Quality Primary Care?" *Journal of General Internal Medicine* 22, no. 10 (2007): 1385–92.

27. L. Casalino, A. November, R. Berenson, and H. Pham, "Hospitals and Doctors: Hospital-Physician Relations: Two Tracks and the Decline of the Voluntary Medical Staff Model,"*Health Affairs* 27, no. 5 (2008): 1305–14.

28. McCarthy and Mueller, *Community Care of North Carolina*; B. Steiner, A. Denham, E. Ashkin, W. Newton, and others, "Community Care of North Carolina: Improving Care Through Community Health Networks,"*Annals of Family Medicine* 6, no. 4 (2008): 361–67.

29. A. Gawande, "The Cost Conundrum Redux: What a Texas Town Can Teach Us About Health Care," *New Yorker*, June 23, 2009, http://www.newyorker.com/reporting/2009/06/01/090601fa_fact_gawande.

30. J. Robinson and L. Casalino, "Vertical Integration and Organizational Networks in Healthcare,"*Health Affairs* 15, no. 1 (1996): 7–22.

31. Casalino and others, "External Incentives, Information Technology, and Organized Processes to Improve Health Care Quality for Patients with Chronic Diseases"; Rittenhouse and Robinson, "Improving Quality in Medicaid."

32. Robinson and Casalino, "Vertical Integration and Organizational Networks in Healthcare."

33. Pittsburgh Regional Health Initiative, *Account Care Networks: Transitions for Small Practices and Community Hospitals* (Pittsburgh, PA: Pittsburgh Regional Health Initiative/Jewish Healthcare Foundation, August 2009), http://prhi.org/docs/Accountable%20Care%20%20Networks.pdf.

34. Fisher and others, "Variations in the Longitudinal Efficiency of Academic Medical Centers"; Fisher and others, "The Implications of Regional Variations in Medicare Spending."Part 1.

35. E. Fisher, M. McClellan, J. Bertko and others, "Fostering Accountable Healthcare: Moving Forward in Medicare." *Health Affairs*, 28w219–w231, January 29, 2009.

36. Fisher and others, "Fostering Accountable Health Care."

37. Rittenhouse and others, "Measuring the Medical Home Infrastructure in Large Medical Groups"; Rittenhouse and Shortell, "The Patient-Centered Medical Home."

38. Pittsburgh Regional Health Initiative, *Account Care Networks*.

39. K. Grumbach and J. Mold, "A Health Care Cooperative Extension Service: Transforming Primary Care and Community Health," *JAMA* 301, no. 24 (2009): 2589–91.

40. Centers for Medicare and Medicaid Services, U.S. Department of Health and Human Services, "Medicare Physicians Group Practice Demonstration," 2008, http://www.cms.hhs.gov/DemoProjectsEvalRpts/downloads/PGP_Fact_Sheet.pdf.

CHAPTER FOUR

ACHIEVING THE VISION

Payment Reform

Stuart Guterman
Anthony Shih

Introduction

As noted in previous chapters, the U.S. health care system is generally characterized by fragmentation. To achieve improved quality and efficiency, the health care system must become more organized, including integration between hospitals and physicians—as well as other types of providers in other settings.[1] However, the current predominantly fee-for-service payment system does not promote integration, but rather fosters the fragmentation that we observe. Financial incentives are an important factor in our fragmented delivery system, both encouraging adverse behavior and preventing improvements, because of what is paid for and not paid for and how payment is made. Better alignment between payment methods and the organization and output we desire from our delivery system is required if our health system is to achieve a higher level of performance, with more appropriate, effective, and efficient care.

This chapter begins by reviewing how the evolution of payment methods and other market factors have affected the traditional hospital-medical staff model. This review is followed by a discussion of payment methodologies that are viewed as potentially useful in appropriately aligning hospital and physician incentives with the patient's best interest. The conclusion outlines the authors'

The views presented are those of the authors and should not be attributed to The Commonwealth Fund, IPRO, their directors, or their officers.

own recommendations for payment reform—offering providers along the continuum of integration alternative payment methods, with the ultimate goal of encouraging greater integration and rewarding higher quality and efficiency.

Evolution of Payment Methods and the Hospital-Physician Relationship

Over the years, the relationship between hospitals and physicians has changed, along with the way both hospitals and physicians are paid. In 1980 Mark Pauly described the hospital as the "doctor's workshop"—providing a setting and inputs into the provision of health care, which physicians oversaw as the agent of the patient.[2] By that time, however, the role of the hospital already had been changing: in 1965 before Medicare and Medicaid made hospital care more accessible to the elderly (and later the disabled) and the poor, respectively, hospital services accounted for 40 percent of personal health care; by 1980, that share was 47 percent.[3] Hospitals' share of the total health care bill peaked in 1982 at 48 percent. Physician spending, which had been 60 percent as great as hospital spending in 1965, had fallen to 45 percent as great by 1982.

This was a period of tremendous innovation in health care technology, combined with increased access to those services provided by an expansion of third-party payment—public and private insurance, which had accounted for 25 percent of all personal health care spending in 1965, had ballooned to 54 percent by 1982. Hospitals were no longer merely doctors' workshops, but the hub of the health care delivery system, and that system was growing rapidly: national health expenditures, equal to 5.9 percent of the gross domestic product (GDP) in 1965, had grown to 10.2 percent of GDP by 1982.

Much of the impetus for the increase in health spending during this period came from the method of payment. When Medicare began in 1966, it adopted the approach used by many private insurance carriers, particularly the Blue Cross and Blue Shield plans who were retained to do most of the claims processing and bill paying for the program. Hospitals were retrospectively reimbursed for the *reasonable costs* they incurred in providing covered services to Medicare patients. Physicians were paid a fee based on *usual, customary, and reasonable charges*, meaning that they received whatever they charged, up to a limit based on the distribution of charges for each service in each local area.[4] Neither of these payment methods provided any incentive for cost containment. Hospitals were reimbursed essentially all the costs they incurred (subject to the exclusion, by definition, of certain categories of costs), and physicians were paid essentially whatever they charged for whatever services they provided; the more providers did, the more they were paid. Quality (which was rarely, if ever, explicitly measured and almost never publicly disclosed) was not a factor in determining the amount of payment, either for hospitals or physicians.

One by-product of this payment environment was that there was very little cause for conflict between hospitals and physicians. Both were paid more for treating more patients and for providing them with more—and more expensive— services. Incentives essentially were aligned across the two groups—but not in favor of more appropriate, effective, and efficient care.

The resulting situation was not sustainable. As health care spending rose rapidly, private insurance premiums increased faster than workers' incomes, putting pressure on both employers and employees, and threatening the competitiveness of American businesses as well as access to and affordability of health coverage. Medicare and Medicaid spending took up an increasing portion of the federal budget, putting pressure on both the budget and the viability of those and other public programs. In 1982 Medicare's actuaries projected that the Hospital Insurance Trust Fund—the source of funding for Medicare's hospital inpatient and other institution-based services, financed out of a dedicated payroll tax paid by almost all workers (and their employers)—would become insolvent by 1987, or within five years.[5]

Medicare Prospective Payment: The First Major Step Toward Bundled Payment

Faced with the imminent insolvency of the Health Insurance Trust Fund, Congress acted to constrain the growth of Medicare hospital spending. In the Tax Equity and Fiscal Responsibility Act of 1982 (TEFRA), they imposed temporary limits on hospital payments and required the Secretary of the Department of Health and Human Services to develop a plan for prospective payment, under which a price would be set in advance for each type of patient. This plan was delivered to Congress in December 1982, and the Medicare Prospective Payment System (PPS) for hospital inpatient services was enacted in April 1983 (as part of the Social Security Amendments of 1983). The new system was implemented beginning on October 1 of that year.

Under the Medicare PPS, each hospital patient is assigned to a *diagnosis-related group* (DRG), depending on the patient's clinical condition and severity, and price is set to represent the relative costliness of patients in each DRG.[6] The price paid to each hospital for each case is fixed. If the hospital can keep its cost below that level, it retains the difference; if the cost for the case exceeds the payment rate, the hospital is expected to offset the resulting shortfall with net revenues from lower-cost cases.[7] With this change from retrospective cost reimbursement to prospective payment for each case, the incentives facing hospitals changed dramatically: the unit of payment changed from the service to the case, which focused broader attention on the treatment of the patient (at least while the patient is in the hospital), and higher costs no longer meant higher payments, so the ability to control the cost of each case directly affected the hospital's financial status.

The implementation of prospective payment apparently succeeded in slowing the growth of Medicare hospital spending: by 1988, the projected insolvency date for the Hospital Insurance Trust Fund had receded to 2005, or seventeen years in the future.[8] It also, however, changed the relationship between hospitals and physicians: by putting pressure on the hospital to control the cost of each case, the new payment system put the hospital in potential conflict with the physician, who, as the agent for the patient and given the prevailing physician payment system, would have the incentive to order more, rather than fewer, services during the stay.

Two other potential areas of divergence arose between the hospital and the physicians who treat patients there: although payment on a per admission basis creates an incentive for the hospital to generate more admissions, the physician does not necessarily realize an increase in payment from additional admissions, depending on what services are provided during the additional stay and whether those services are provided by the admitting physician or another physician. In addition, the fixed payment per stay creates the incentive for the hospital to discharge patients earlier—because, other things being equal, earlier discharge keeps the hospital's costs down while having no effect on its payment—although that could be expected to meet resistance from the patient and the patient's physician. In fact, the lack of incentive for physicians to increase the number of admissions appears to have played a role in keeping hospital volume from increasing as feared with the implementation of the PPS.[9] Moreover, conflicts between physicians and hospitals over early discharge created a controversy over "quicker and sicker" discharges—that is, the allegation that hospitals were pressuring physicians to discharge their patients prematurely.[10]

In the years immediately following the implementation of Medicare prospective payment, a number of Medicaid programs and private insurers followed suit with similar case-based programs. In 1994 the U.S. Department of Health and Human services reported that "about two-thirds of Blue Cross and Blue Shield plans surveyed use Medicare's prospective hospital payment approach for at least one of their plans covering hospital services. Moreover, 21 states use a similar approach for their Medicaid program."[11] Although many payers may since have adopted different payment methods, their payment rates often are pegged to Medicare rates. This keeps the pressure on the relationship between hospitals and physicians.

Resource-Based Relative Value Scale: Revising Prices for Individual Physician Services

After the relatively successful implementation of the Medicare prospective payment system for hospital inpatient services, attention turned to physician payment. Although it had been growing more slowly than hospital spending, physician spending nonetheless had been rapidly increasing, from $8.3 billion in 1965 to

$60.8 billion in 1982—an annual rate of increase of 12.4 percent. Moreover, while hospital spending had increased faster than physician spending in fourteen of the seventeen years since Medicare had begun, physician spending began to grow faster than hospital spending after the implementation of the 1982 TEFRA limits on hospital spending and then PPS payment in 1983.[12]

After some consideration of using DRGs to calculate physician payments as well as hospital payments, Congress, in the Omnibus Budget Reconciliation Act of 1989 (OBRA89), replaced the charge-based payment system that had been used (with some adjustments) since Medicare's inception in 1966 with a physician fee schedule.[13] This new rate-setting mechanism, which went into effect in January 1992, was intended to address several objectives.[14] First, it based payment for each service on an estimate of the resources required to provide it (the resource-based relative value scale, or RBRVS), rather than each physician's own charges for the services. This methodology was intended to reduce price variation across physicians and geographic areas (while accounting for differences in practice costs) and to slow charge inflation and spending growth. Second, the relative values were used to correct what was perceived to be a distortion in the charge structure, which had led to a growing gap between payments for evaluation and management and those for surgeries and procedures. This gap was thought to exceed differences in the costs of providing these services, encouraging increasing numbers of more complex, invasive, and expensive services. Third, because the physician has more or less direct control over the volume and mix of services provided, the new mechanism included a component that responded to overall increases in volume and intensity by reducing prices, in order to reduce the growth in total physician spending. As in the case of Medicare hospital payment—and perhaps to an even greater degree—the RBRVS methodology was adopted and has continued to be used by many Medicaid programs, as well as private payers.[15]

Several criticisms have been leveled at the Medicare physician fee schedule. Although the RBRVS initially reduced the distortion in fees that favored surgeries and procedures relative to evaluation and management, two major trends have led to a reappearance and growth of that distortion: the development of expensive new procedures over time and what many describe as a specialty-dominated process for revising the relative weights that determine the distribution of payments across services. As a result of these trends, many stakeholders became concerned about the role of the RBRVS in encouraging both the increasing numbers of procedures and imaging and the diminishing role of primary care.[16] Moreover, the Sustainable Growth Rate (SGR) mechanism, which has been used since 1998 to determine the annual increase in physician fees based on actual cumulative physician spending relative to a target, has produced a succession of cuts in response to the fact that actual spending has exceeded the target since 2002.[17]

Although Congress has intervened to avoid reductions in Medicare physician fees every year since 2003, the attempt to control physician spending growth—which is driven primarily by the volume and intensity of services—by ratcheting down on the price of services across the board has put more pressure on the payment system and exacerbated the effects of the distortions in relative prices. This pressure has made it more difficult to align incentives properly, both among physicians and across settings. Also, because Congress often looks to offset the cost of avoiding the annual physician fee cuts by finding savings from other provider payments, this process has pitted physicians against hospitals and other types of providers in determining the distribution of scarce funding.

Managed Care as a Model for Aligning Financial Incentives

Many experts believe that *managed care* provides a model for aligning the financial incentives of hospitals and physicians. To some extent, the rise of managed care did lead to the creation of innovative physician hospital organizations designed to give these providers better negotiating power with managed care plans. This development had the side effect of aligning hospital and physician incentives—although there is some debate about whether that alignment produced higher quality, or even more efficient, care. In any case, the retreat from managed care in the late 1990s essentially stopped the development of such organizations.

Managed care in its original form evolved beginning around 1930 as a way to provide organized health care to select groups of people in communities around the country.[18] By providing health care to its members for a prepaid fee, the managed care plan was able to ensure the availability and accessibility of care. Because the fee was fixed, the plan had a strong incentive to provide effective care in a cost-efficient manner. As these prepaid health plans evolved, there was increasing emphasis on preventive care and other ways of maintaining members' health, giving rise to the term *health maintenance organizations* (HMOs). The prepaid health plan model was not met with great enthusiasm by the medical establishment, as it was a perceived as a threat to their clinical autonomy and their income. As noted by Fox and Kongstvedt, "In 1932 the American Medical Association (AMA) adopted a strong stance against prepaid group practices, favoring instead indemnity type insurance."[19] Because managing care appropriately could be expected to reduce hospital admissions, the hospital industry was not an early supporter of this model either.

The Committee on the Cost of Medical Care, an influential group of medical and economic experts convened in the early 1930s to address the rising cost of health care, nonetheless recommended expansion of the prepaid group practice model as a way of addressing health care inflation.[20] In the 1930s and 1940s, despite opposition from many physicians and hospitals, some of the best-known managed care organizations—the Kaiser Foundation Health Plan in Southern California, the Group Health Association in Washington, D.C., the Health Insurance Plan of Greater New York, and the Group Health Cooperative of Puget Sound in Seattle, Washington—began operating.[21] These organizations differed in their corporate structures, but they all focused on comprehensive and coordinated health care. By the 1950s, prepayment plans had established a small but stable niche in the health care sector. Their payment methods generally did not spread beyond a small number of staff and group model health care organizations to affect the larger provider community. However, concern about protecting their patient base against competition from Kaiser did lead the San Joaquin County, California, Medical Society to form the San Joaquin Medical Foundation, which accepted capitated payments from subscribers and paid the affiliated independent physicians and hospitals according to a relative value–based fee schedule. This is considered the earliest example of the *independent practice association* (IPA) model.[22]

With renewed interest in rising health care spending nationwide in the late 1960s and early 1970s, attention became focused on managed care as a potential vehicle for providing better care at lower cost. In 1971 the Nixon Administration announced that HMOs were to be part of a new national health strategy.[23] Congress subsequently passed the Health Maintenance Organization Act of 1973, which defined HMOs, provided grants and loans for the start-up of nonprofit HMOs, and required all employers of twenty-five or more employees to offer at least one prepaid group practice and one IPA as health insurance options wherever they were available and requested to be offered.[24] This legislation, and the inclusion of an option for Medicare beneficiaries to enroll in HMOs, supported the growth of prepaid health plans—and the development of variations on this model—through the 1970s and 1980s. By 1985, there were almost 20 million HMO enrollees, and by 1992, there were almost 40 million.[25] With the growth of the managed care model, however, variants on the original HMO had become a bigger part of the market: the traditional staff- and group-model HMOs, which had accounted for 57 percent of HMO enrollees in 1985, accounted for only 31 percent of HMO enrollees in 1992; 59 percent of HMO enrollees were in IPA and mixed-model HMOs.

One of the major changes that also occurred during the late 1980s and early 1990s was a separation in many plans of the financing and delivery aspects of the plan's functions. This change set up increasingly adversarial relationships between the health plans and providers, and among providers, including hospitals and physicians. Notably, this trend increasingly pitted patients (and many of their providers) against the plans, as they perceived their access to desired services to be threatened by referral requirements and coverage denials (see the following discussion).

During the height of managed care in the mid-1990s, physicians began to aggregate into larger multispecialty groups, IPAs, or physician hospital organizations. Physicians hoped that such aggregation would achieve economies of scale, allow them to take advantage of the referral benefits of having primary care physicians within the organization, and create negotiating leverage with health plans.

Although the general population reported fairly high levels of satisfaction under managed care, those with chronic illnesses (with greater exposure to utilization management) were much less satisfied with their care, compared with the prior fee-for-service environment.[26] However, satisfaction varied with factors such as ownership status (nonprofit versus for-profit) and plan type (staff model versus discounted fee-for-service).[27] By the late 1990s, initial consumer support for managed care—particularly in its more restrictive forms—had declined as people worried that needed care might be withheld and wanted greater control over the health care options available to them. Researchers found that patients in managed care plans valued their primary care provider's role as care coordinators, but wanted them to refrain from acting as gatekeepers to specialty care.[28] Employees and their employers began to demand broad, almost universal choice among providers. This backlash resulted in marketplace, legislative, and legal reactions that altered the operations of most managed care organizations and HMOs. Managed care enrollment peaked in 1999 at about 80 million—after rapid growth throughout the decade—and fell back under 70 million by 2004.

As managed care organizations and health plans reduced cost containment restrictions to try to stem the exodus of enrollees, large multispecialty groups, IPAs, and physician hospital organizations lost many of the advantages that had brought them together in the mid-1990s. Physicians became more distant from hospitals, and many stopped providing services they had provided traditionally, including emergency department call and service on hospital committees.[29]

Even in the case of managed care, then, forces both internal and external to the market have conspired to counteract the potential for alignment of financial incentives between hospitals and physicians—and, most importantly, failed to produce consistent support for the achievement of high quality and efficiency of care across settings.

Moving Toward New Incentives

As concerns continue to grow regarding the quality and cost of care, a variety of payment reforms are being discussed and tested that may directly affect hospital reimbursement and potentially affect the hospital-physician relationship. These range from modifications of payment that can be built on a fee-for-service (FFS) framework to more comprehensive payment approaches that move further away from the current system. The following section reviews some of the leading proposals, focusing on their impact on the hospital-physician relationship, their likely impact on quality and efficiency, and some key implementation issues. The main points are summarized in Table 4.1.

TABLE 4.1 LEADING PAYMENT PROPOSALS THAT AFFECT THE HOSPITAL-PHYSICIAN RELATIONSHIP

Payment Method	Alignment with Quality and Efficiency	Impact on Hospital-Physician Relationship	Key Implementation Issues
Pay-for-performance (provider- or group-specific).	Promotes quality; difficult to construct to promote efficiency.	Hospitals incentivized to work with physicians on inpatient care only. No incentive for physicians to work with hospitals.	Relatively easy to implement (already widespread).
Shared savings: physicians share savings for a defined group of patients.	Promotes efficiency; can add quality incentives to payment.	Physicians incentivized to coordinate care with hospitals (especially to reduce readmissions) but not vice versa; incentives to reduce hospitalizations may aggravate hospital-physician relationship.	Difficult to calculate savings.
Shared savings: physicians and hospitals share savings for a defined group of patients.	Promotes efficiency; can add quality incentives to payment.	Hospitals and physicians incentivized to coordinate care; depending on hospital share of savings payments, incentives to reduce hospitalizations may aggravate hospital-physician relationship.	Difficult to calculate savings; creates payment allocation issues among providers.
Acute care episode payment: extend hospital DRG payment to postacute period; exclude physician and other services.	Promotes efficiency within the episode but does not control number of episodes; can add quality incentives to payment.	Hospitals incentivized to coordinate care with physicians; no incentive for physicians to work with hospitals.	Among episode-based payments, relatively easy to implement.
Acute care episode payment: include hospital and physician services (and potentially other) services.	Promotes efficiency within the episode but does not control number of episodes; can add quality incentives to payment.	Hospital and physicians incentivized to coordinate care, but both parties must share a fixed dollar amount.	Difficult to construct payment; creates payment allocation issues between physicians and hospitals.

Payment type			
Chronic care episode payment (physician care only).	Promotes efficiency within the episode but does not control number of episodes;can add quality incentives to payment.	No strong incentive to coordinate care between hospitals and physicians; incentives to reduce hospitalizations may aggravate hospital-physician relationship.	Difficult to construct payment, especially with multiple comorbid conditions.
Chronic care episode payment: including physician and hospital (and potentially other) services.	Promotes efficiency within the episode but does not control number of episodes; can add quality incentives to payment.	Hospitals and physicians incentivized to coordinate care, but both parties must share a fixed dollar amount.	Difficult to construct payment, especially with multiple comorbid conditions; creates payment allocation issues between physicians and hospitals.
Blended payment for primary care (for example, medical home payment).	Promotes coordinated care and quality; does not directly promote efficiency.	No strong incentive to coordinate care between hospitals and physicians; incentives to reduce hospitalizations may aggravate hospital-physician relationship.	Primary implementation issue is qualifying providers for payment; several public and private demonstrations under way.
Capitation: global per patient fee including all services.	Promotes efficiency; can add quality incentives to payment.	Hospitals and physicians incentivized to coordinate care, but both parties must share a fixed dollar amount.	Strong incentives for patient selection; carving out certain services likely to reduce efficiency; payment allocation issues among providers.

Source: Authors' analysis.

Pay-for-Performance

One of the more straightforward payment reform strategies for hospitals is referred to as *pay-for-performance* (P4P). In its current form, this approach involves awarding bonuses to providers, in addition to their payments under the current FFS system, for high scores on a specified set of quality measures. Pay-for-performance is intended to serve two purposes: first, it sends a signal through the payment system that the system will reward high quality, rather than merely high volume and intensity; second, it focuses attention on a set of specific metrics that have been defined as representing high quality, providing information for providers as to how that term is defined by payers.

Representative of this approach is the Medicare Hospital Quality Incentive (HQI) Demonstration being conducted by the Centers for Medicare and Medicaid Services (CMS). Under this demonstration, participating hospitals, in addition to their normal reimbursement under the PPS system, are eligible to receive bonuses based on their performance on quality measures for patients admitted for heart attack, heart failure, pneumonia, coronary artery bypass graft, and hip and knee replacements.[30] This demonstration began in 2003 at about the same time that all hospitals began reporting (much more limited) data on quality indicators to CMS. An early evaluation found that hospitals engaged in this demonstration achieved modestly greater improvements in quality (at least among the common measures available) than hospitals engaged only in public reporting.[31]

Concern about this approach has been raised on two fronts. First, critics of pay-for-performance—at least in its current state of development—note that most applications of P4P focus on structure and process measures (such as the availability of health information technology or the administration of appropriate medication to patients with a specific condition), rather than patient outcomes. Second, there is skepticism about whether the relatively small rewards available under current pay-for-performance initiatives are enough to counteract the much larger adverse incentives presented by the current fee-for-service payment system. These concerns are well taken, but they do not obviate the need to incorporate explicit rewards for high quality into the way health care is paid for. Also, the use of pay-for-performance approaches has even more potential value as alternatives to fee-for-service payment are developed and implemented, and as measures are refined and data to populate them improved.

Another form of pay-for-performance is the recently implemented CMS payment policy of not providing additional payments for certain complications that were not present on admission, or *never events*.[32] This approach, as currently in effect, affects only a minute share of Medicare hospital payments, but it apparently has generated a great deal of response on the part of hospitals, with the prospect that it may be applied to a broader set of conditions in the future. It is an example of the "stick"—that is, a negative incentive to avoid quality problems—along with the "carrot" represented by the more traditional pay-for-performance approach used in the HQI demonstration.

In both of these examples, the payment system offers a financial incentive related to the quality of care, with no direct consideration of the efficiency with which that care is provided (that is, beyond the incentives for efficiency at the level of the hospital stay that DRG payment provides). Moreover, these and most programs like them focus on measures of hospital performance that relate solely to care delivered in the hospital. Therefore, although they create an incentive for hospitals to work more closely with the physicians practicing in the hospital, they do not create an incentive for hospital-physician collaboration or coordination of patient care outside of the hospital setting. Further, because payments are made directly to the hospitals, and not to physicians practicing in them, hospital and physician financial incentives are not strongly aligned.

Similar pay-for-performance approaches are being developed and tested in both the private and public sectors for application to physician services. However, the state of the art in measuring physician quality (for most specialties) is not as well developed as it is for the hospital setting, and concerns have been raised about the ability to measure quality and structure corresponding financial rewards for individual physicians. Work continues on this front, and the potential for grouping physicians (and perhaps other providers) for the purpose of quality measurement and rewards is attracting interest.[33]

Work also is being done to develop measures of performance for application to health care at the system level, but this effort is considerably more difficult even than the development of provider-specific measures. When such measures are ready for application, they will be useful in emphasizing the importance of coordinated care across providers and settings, rather than the fragmented health care that typifies the current system.

Shared Savings

It is important to reward efficient care as well as high quality. But using measures of efficiency in pay-for-performance initiatives such as those described earlier may distort incentives and fail to establish an explicit connection between the amount of savings and the size of the reward. This issue is addressed in part by reforms that explicitly include shared savings payments to reward efficiency, such as the Physician Group Practice (PGP) demonstration initiated by Medicare in 2005 in ten large multispecialty group practices. In the PGP demonstration, participants are not only rewarded for better outpatient care as defined by performance on quality of care measures, but are also eligible to "share" some of the savings from better overall cost control, largely from reduced hospitalization rates. In the third year of the demonstration, five of the ten participating physician group practices had slowed the growth in Medicare expenditures for their patients enough to qualify for performance payments for cost efficiency.[34] An interesting feature of this demonstration is that 50 percent of the bonus payment pool generated by each practice's efficiency relative to its spending target is distributed on the basis of quality improvement metrics specified in advance. An alternative approach would be to create a bonus pool for high performance on quality measures (for example, by setting aside a proportion of the base payment rates), which can be supplemented by any savings that result from increased efficiency.

The ability of shared savings model to incentivize hospital-physician collaboration depends greatly on how and with whom the savings are shared. If the payment model is used for physicians groups that are not part of integrated delivery systems with hospitals, hospitals can't share in the savings and are not incentivized to work with the physicians (in fact, it can be quite the opposite, as the savings for which physicians are rewarded are expected to come largely from reduced hospitalizations). Therefore, to promote hospital-physician collaboration, shared savings must explicitly reward hospitals for savings, or be applied to organizational forms such as integrated delivery systems.

Major challenges to the implementation of shared savings approaches include determining the patient population for which the providers are to be responsible and the spending target to which their performance is to be compared, and calculating the savings generated. One approach would hold providers or groups of providers responsible for patients who enroll with them (with perhaps a financial reward for patients who do so). Another, used in the Medicare PGP demonstration, would use administrative data to empirically assign patients to the provider organization to be paid.[35] That is, they wouldn't have to *enroll* with the organization, but would be assigned for shared savings payment purposes to an organization based on their past utilization. In contrast to the PGP demonstration, which used comparison groups, Fisher and colleagues proposed a model that would use historical data to project cost growth rates for beneficiaries in order to benchmark costs for the purpose of the shared savings calculations. This approach was developed for application to *accountable care organizations* (ACOs).[36] As described in the previous chapter, these would be entities that could be clinically and fiscally accountable for the entire continuum of care that patients might need, and could be organized in various forms, such as integrated delivery systems, multispecialty group practices, or physician hospital organizations.

Blended Payment for Primary Care

One of the more prominent payment reforms currently under discussion involves a specific organizational structure in primary care—the *patient-centered medical home*. In early 2007, the American Academy of Family Physicians, the American Academy of Pediatrics, the American College of Physicians, and the American Osteopathic Association issued joint principles for the patient-centered medical home, an approach to providing comprehensive primary care to children, youth, and adults.[37] There is ample evidence that a greater emphasis on primary care is associated with better health outcomes and lower costs.[38] One of the joint principles is a payment system that recognizes the additional services and value of the medical home, including care coordination, health information technology, enhanced communication, and remote monitoring. There are currently dozens of private payer pilots across the country, as well as a large Medicare Medical Home Demonstration project underway.

Although the specifics of each demonstration vary, they virtually all include an enhanced payment for medical home practices, usually in the form of a per member per month *care management fee*, in addition to traditional fee-for-service payments for face-to-face encounters. Payers have agreed to this approach in the hopes of long-term cost savings, particularly due to lower hospitalization costs, as reported in the Geisinger experience, and in analogous experiences with similar primary care case management programs.[39] Although this payment model applies to ambulatory care, it impacts the hospital-physician relationship because it increases the financial tensions between independent hospitals and outpatient providers, who are working in part to keep their patients outside of the hospital setting.

One of the key challenges of implementing this payment model is qualifying practices to be eligible to receive such payment. Although the payment model does not require that there be a hospital-physician relationship, as bundled episode payments do (see the following discussion), it does require that practices have an infrastructure that most current small practices don't have, such as health information technology, access twenty-four hours a day and seven days a week, and capabilities for care management. Thus more widespread adoption of this model may incentivize small physician practices to form or join larger groups, which can provide or assist with the infrastructure requirements. For instance, larger groups are more than twice as likely as small physician practices to use electronic health records.[40]

Episode-Based Payment Strategies

Broadly defined, an *episode-based payment* is a payment for services for the care of a patient during a period of time (longer than a single visit or hospitalization). In contrast to the fee-for-service system, which rewards volume and fosters fragmentation of the delivery system, episode-based payments have the potential to encourage care coordination and efficiency.[41] There are numerous variations on how this might be done, but it is useful for discussion to identify four broad categories:

- Payment for acute care episodes (that is, services triggered by or built around a hospitalization and extending for a period beyond the hospitalization) that include hospital services only
- Payment for acute care episodes that include both hospital and physician services (and potentially other services as well)
- Payment for chronic care episodes (for example, diabetes care for one year) that include outpatient care only
- Payment for chronic care episodes that include outpatient plus inpatient care (and potentially other services as well)

Each of these variations has a different impact on the alignment of hospital and physician clinical and financial services, as well as on incentives for coordination of inpatient and outpatient care. The most straightforward extension of the current payment system to episode-based payment would be the extension of DRG payments to hospitals to include a period, such as thirty days, following discharge from an initial hospitalization. This type of bundled payment would strongly incentivize hospitals to improve care coordination and the transition from hospital to outpatient care (or home), as they would be at risk for readmissions related to the original hospitalization within the thirty-day period, as well as emergency room visits. If the bundle included only inpatient care, however, although hospitals would have the incentive to work with the outpatient community, other providers would have little financial incentive to reciprocate. If, however, the episode payment included both hospital and physician services in the bundle, then both parties would be financially incentivized to coordinate care. This latter approach presents several significant challenges. In addition to the difficulty of constructing the total payment amount, it requires a method to allocate and distribute the payments among hospitals and physicians, which is particularly difficult in the context of the current fragmented health care system. Such payments appear to be feasible only under a structure such as a physician hospital organization, an integrated delivery system, or other accountable care organization (see Chapter Three for a description of alternative ACO models).

Geisinger ProvenCare is one example of an acute episode-based payment system developed by an integrated delivery system. A single payment for a ProvenCare coronary artery bypass graft (CABG) covers preoperative evaluation and workup, all hospital and professional fees, all routine postdischarge care, and management of any related complications within ninety days of the CABG surgery (including readmissions).[42] In this system, there is a strong incentive for both hospitals and physicians to deliver high-quality, coordinated care, as they are at risk for the cost of complications. Although sharing a fixed payment creates competing financial incentives among providers, this is addressed in the Geisinger case because they are an integrated delivery system, with existing infrastructure for allocating resources. It may be that episode-based payment systems stimulate greater integration of hospital and physician services because of this issue.

PROMETHEUS Payment is a new episode-based payment system that does not require that payment be made to a single integrated organization. The payments, called *evidence-informed case rates*, are severity adjusted, and they are derived from the resources required to deliver care as recommended with the best available clinical evidence, with an allowance for potentially avoidable complications.[43] Although the case rates cover the cost of care for an entire episode, the payment does not require prospective payment. In current pilots, providers are reimbursed fee-for-service and are reconciled against the case budgets on a quarterly basis.[44] In the design of the system, there is also a performance withhold for quality, efficiency, and patient satisfaction. However, because part of the withhold depends on the performance of the entire care team during the episode (that is, inpatient and outpatient care), both hospitals and physicians, even when not members of the same organizational structure, both share financial incentives to deliver the best care. This new payment system is currently undergoing pilot testing and has not been fully evaluated yet.

In addition to the implementation challenges of acute episode-based payments that bundle hospital and physician services, there are other significant concerns. First, although an episode-based payment incentivizes efficient delivery of services within the episode, there is no control of the volume of episodes. To the contrary, there is an incentive to increase the number of episodes (in this respect, it is similar to a fee-for-service payment system). Second, although the hope is that episode-based payment systems foster more organized delivery systems, it may be that they instead foster the creation of multiple condition-specific hospital-physician service units. To the extent that these units are focused on treating specific conditions, rather than meeting the broader medical needs of their patients, there may be paradoxically increased fragmentation of care delivery.

Episode-based payments for chronic conditions have generated less discussion than acute episode-based payment systems. Compared with acute episode-based payments, they face the additional challenges of defining the beginning and end of an episode. In addition, the nature of ambulatory care is to focus on multiple chronic conditions, meaning that a single patient may qualify for multiple chronic episode payments. Similar to the acute episode-based payments, the chronic episode-based payments that bundle both physician and hospital care incentivize coordination between the two parties, but also face the problems of payment allocation and distribution. Likewise, a payment system that includes only physician services incentivizes physicians to coordinate with hospitals, but not vice versa. Further, the general issue of volume control in episode-based payments is exacerbated in chronic care, as it is likely easier for a provider to qualify a patient for a chronic care episode than an acute one, making it that much easier for providers to generate more and more episodes.

Capitation, or Global Payment

Full capitation, or global per member, per month payment, would strongly incentivize efficiency and coordination between hospital and physicians. In addition, with the appropriate pay-for-performance quality incentives in place, it would also be aligned with better quality and protect against underutilization. Further, unlike bundled episode payments, there is no opportunity to increase revenue by increasing volume. However, unless payment is adequately adjusted for patients who are more or less likely than average to incur high expenses, there is a strong incentive for providers to try to attract healthy patients and avoid sick ones—a problem that caused great concern during the peak of managed care enrollment in the 1990s. Attempts to address this issue by carving out certain services from the global payment may decrease the incentive for providers to be efficient.

Similar to other payment strategies that bundle hospital, physician, and other provider services together, this strategy creates payment allocation issues among the providers, who are competing for a fixed dollar amount. Successful implementation is therefore most likely in the more highly organized structures, such as integrated delivery systems and large, multispecialty group practices. Kaiser Permanente is a large integrated delivery system in California that provides one example of how a global payment mechanism is applied to align incentives across all the providers who are responsible for a group of patients (in this case, Kaiser members).

Conclusion

As consumers of health care, we want our health care delivery system to provide high-quality, efficient care. In the United States, achieving this goal is complicated by the fragmentation of the delivery system and a payment structure that primarily rewards volume and intensity, creating competing incentives among providers. Many of the payment solutions being discussed and tested may effectively align provider performance with health care system quality and efficiency. However, they may also exacerbate tensions between physicians and hospitals, particularly if cost savings are achieved through reduced hospitalizations. These tensions can be mitigated with greater organizational integration of physicians and hospitals (see Chapter Three). Greater integration would likewise enable providers to deliver higher quality, more efficient care.[45] Payment, organizational structure, and health care delivery are closely linked; and they must be considered simultaneously. If the health care system is to deliver high-quality, efficient care, not only should the payment system reward quality and efficiency but it should also stimulate the organizational structures that allow the delivery of high-quality, efficient care.

Acknowledging that the health care system cannot jump immediately to a global payment model that only integrated delivery systems can effectively implement, we propose that payers adopt a flexible payment approach—one that offers an array of alternative payment models that incentivize quality and efficiency through various levels of payment reforms, matched to the capabilities of the current organizational structures.[46] For example, payers might offer a blended fee-for-service and care management fee payment model for practices that are able to meet the requirements of the medical home model, a global DRG case rate model that includes hospital and postacute care for formal or informal systems that can accept responsibility for patients across the continuum of care during and following an inpatient stay, and a global payment per enrollee for more organized systems. This is depicted in Figure 4.1.

FIGURE 4.1   A FLEXIBLE PAYMENT APPROACH

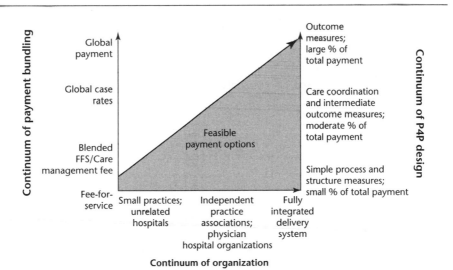

Source: Adapted from A. Shih, K. Davis, S. Schoenbaum, A. Gauthier, and others, *Organizing the U.S. Health Care Delivery System for High Performance* (New York: The Commonwealth Fund, 2008), Exhibit ES-1, p. xi.

This model would have greater potential financial rewards for quality and efficiency the more bundled the payment and coordinated the care. For instance, the medical home payment model might have 5 percent bonuses tied to quality-based incentives, whereas the global payment might have 20 percent bonuses. More bundled payments also already reward more efficient care delivery. As only more integrated systems would be more likely to succeed under the more-bundled payment models, this approach would incentivize the gradual integration—either actual or virtual—of providers.

For this payment model to succeed, a more coordinated strategy between public and private payers needs to be developed and implemented. We would encourage that all payers consider this type of flexible payment approach. Ultimately, the goal is higher performance in the health system, which can only be achieved through better organization of the delivery system, which must be supported by the appropriate financial incentives.

Notes

1. A. Shih, K. Davis, S. C. Schoenbaum, A. Gauthier, and others, *Organizing the U.S. Health Care Delivery System for High Performance* (New York: The Commonwealth Fund, 2008), http://www.commonwealthfund.org/Content/Publications/Fund-Reports/2008/Aug/Organizing-the-U-S--Health-Care-Delivery-System-for-High-Performance.aspx.

2. M. V. Pauly, *Doctors and Their Workshops* (Chicago: University of Chicago Press, 1980).

3. Centers for Medicare and Medicaid Services, "National Health Expenditures Data, 1965–2007,"http://www.cms.hhs.gov/NationalHealthExpendData (accessed June 26, 2009).

4. J. P. Newhouse, "Medicare's Challenges in Paying Providers,"*Health Care Financing Review* 27, no. 2 (Winter 2005–2006): 35–44.

5. M. Moon, "Assessing the Viability of Medicare: Testimony for the Joint Economic Committee" (April 10, 2003), http://www.urban.org/publications/900601.html (accessed June 26, 2009).

6. The price each hospital receives for each patient is also adjusted for local market characteristics that affect the cost of treatment and for the indirect costs of graduate medical education and the hospital's share of Medicaid and low-income Medicare patients.

7. Hospitals receive additional outlier payments for exceptionally expensive cases, but these payments apply only in a small percentage of cases, and hospitals incur a substantial loss on outlier cases before the additional payments begin.

8. Moon, "Assessing the Viability of Medicare."

9. There was enough concern that the incentives in the new payment system would generate more cases that the Congress required the Secretary of Health and Human Services to submit a report on the feasibility of making a volume adjustment or requiring preadmission certification in order to minimize those incentives. See U.S. Department of Health and Human Services, *Report to Congress: Impact of the Medicare Hospital Inpatient Prospective Payment System: 1984 Annual Report* (Baltimore, MD: Health Care Financing Administration, 1986).

10. L. V. Rubenstein, R. H. Brook, D. Draper, W. H. Rogers, and others, "Prospective Payment System and Impairment at Discharge: The 'Quicker and Sicker' Story Revisited," *JAMA* 264, no. 15 (October 17, 1990): 1980–83.

11. U.S. Department of Health and Human Services, "Medicare Payment Methods Used by Private Insurers" (Medicaid press release, September 28, 1994), http://www.hhs.gov/news/press/prel995pres/940928.txt (accessed July 2, 2009).

12. In fact, physician spending grew faster than hospital spending for nineteen consecutive years beginning in 1983, the year TEFRA was implemented. Data from Centers for Medicare and Medicaid Services, "National Health Expenditures Data, 1965–2007."

13. G. R. Wilensky, "Reforming Medicare's Physician Payment System, *New England Journal of Medicine* 360, no. 7 (February 12, 2009): 653–55.

14. M. Miller, "Medicare Payment to Physicians: Testimony Before the Subcommittee on Health, Committee on Energy and Commerce, U.S. House of Representatives, July 26, 2006,"http://www.medpac.gov/publications/congressional_testimony/072506_Testimony_physician.pdf (accessed June 29, 2009).

15. U.S. Department of Health and Human Services, "Medicare Payment Methods Used by Private Insurers."

16. P. B. Ginsburg and R. A. Berenson, "Revising Medicare's Physician Fee Schedule—Much Activity, Little Change," *New England Journal of Medicine* 356, no. 12 (March 22, 2007): 1201–03.

17. Centers for Medicare and Medicaid Services, Office of the Actuary, "Estimated Sustainable Growth Rate and Conversion Factor for Medicare Payments to Physicians in 2009," http://www.cms.hhs.gov/SustainableGRatesConFact/Downloads/sgr2009p.pdf (accessed July 2, 2009).

18. Tufts Managed Care Institute, *A Brief History of Managed Care* (1998), http://thci.org/downloads/BriefHist.pdf (accessed July 3, 2009).

19. P. D. Fox and P. R. Kongstvedt, "The Origins of Managed Health Care," in *Essentials of Managed Health Care*, ed. P. R. Kongstvedt, 5th ed. (Sudbury, MA: Jones & Bartlett, 2007), 4.

20. I. S. Falk, C. R. Rorem, and M. D. Ring, *The Costs of Medical Care: A Summary of Investigations on the Economic Aspects of the Prevention and Care of Illness* (Chicago: University of Chicago Press, 1933).

21. Fox and Kongstvedt, "The Origins of Managed Health Care."

22. Tufts Managed Care Institute, *A Brief History of Managed Care.*

23. Tufts Managed Care Institute, *A Brief History of Managed Care.*

24. A. C. Enthoven and L. Tollen, "Preface," in *Toward a 21st Century Health System*, ed. A. C. Enthoven and L. Tollen, xxvii–xlix (San Francisco: Jossey-Bass, 2004).

25. MCOL, "Managed Care Fact Sheets," http://www.mcareol.com/factshts/factnati.htm (accessed on July 3, 2009).

26. B. G. Druss, M. Schlesinger, T. Thomas, and H. Allen, "Chronic Illness and Plan Satisfaction Under Managed Care," *Health Affairs* 19, no. 6 (January/February 2000): 203–9.

27. C. Schoen and P. Davidson, "Image and Reality: Managed Care Experiences by Plan Type," *Bulletin of the New York Academy of Medicine: Journal of Urban Health* 73 (Winter 1996): S506–S531.

28. K. Grumbach, J. V. Selby, C. Damberg, A. B. Bindman, and others, "Resolving the Gatekeeper Conundrum: What Patients Value in Primary Care and Referrals to Specialists," *JAMA* 282, no. 3 (July 21, 1999): 261–66.

29. R. A. Berenson, P. B. Ginsburg, and J. H. May, "Hospital-Physician Relations: Cooperation, Competition, or Separation?" *Health Affairs* Web exclusive (December 5, 2006), w31–w43, http://content.healthaffairs.org/cgi/content/full/26/1/w31?maxtoshow=&HITS=10&hits=10&RESULTFORMAT=&author1=berenson&andorexactfulltext=and&searchid=1&FIRSTINDEX=0&resourcetype=HWCIT.

30. Centers for Medicare and Medicaid Services, "Premier Hospital Quality Incentive Demonstration" (fact sheet, June 2008), http://www.cms.hhs.gov/HospitalQualityInits/35_hospitalpremier.asp (accessed December 14, 2009).

31. P. K. Lindenaur, D. Remus, S. Roman, M. B. Rothberg, and others, "Public Reporting and Pay for Performance in Hospital Quality Improvement," *New England Journal of Medicine* 356 (2007): 486–96.

32. Centers for Medicare and Medicaid Services, "Hospital Acquired Conditions: Overview,"http://www.cms.hhs.gov/HospitalAcqCond (accessed March 20, 2009).

33. E. S. Fisher, M. B. McClellan, J. Bertko, S. Lieberman, and others, "Fostering Accountable Health Care: Moving Forward in Medicare,"*Health Affairs* Web exclusive (January 27, 2009): w219–w231, http://content.healthaffairs.org/cgi/content/full/28/2/w219?maxtoshow=&HITS=10&hits=10&RESULTFORMAT=&author1=fisher&andorexactfulltext=and&searchid=1&FIRSTINDEX=0&resourcetype=HWCIT.

34. Centers for Medicare and Medicaid Services, "Medicare Physician Group Practice Demonstration" (fact sheet, August 2009), http://www.cms.hhs.gov/DemoProjectsEvalRpts/downloads/PGP_Fact_Sheet.pdf (accessed September 7, 2009).

35. Centers for Medicare and Medicaid Services. "Medicare Physician Group Practice Demonstration,"

36. Fisher and others, "Fostering Accountable Health Care."

37. Patient Centered Primary Care Collaborative, "AAFP, ACP, AOA, AAP: Joint Principles of the Patient Centered Medical Home" (February 2007), http://www.pcpcc.net/node/14 (accessed March 20, 2009).

38. B. Starfield, L. Shi, and J. Macinko, "Contribution of Primary Care to Health Systems and Health,"*Milbank Quarterly* 83, no. 3 (2005): 457–502.

39. R. A. Paulus, K. Davis, and G. D. Steele, "Continuous Innovation in Health Care: Implications of the Geisinger Experience," *Health Affairs* 27, no. 5 (September/October 2008): 1235–45. For the Iowa experience, for example, see E. T. Momany, S. D. Flach, F. D. Nelson, and P. C. Damiano, "A Cost Analysis of the Iowa Medicaid Primary Care Case Management System," *Health Services Research* 41, no. 4, pt. 1 (2006): 1357–71.

40. A. M. Audet, M. M. Doty, J. Shamasdin, and S. C. Schoenbaum, "Measure, Learn, and Improve: Physician's Involvement in Quality Improvement," *Health Affairs* 24, no. 3 (May/June 2005): 843–53.

41. K. Davis, "Paying for Care Episodes and Care Coordination," *New England Journal of Medicine* 356, no. 11 (2007): 1166–68.

42. Paulus and others, "Continuous Innovation in Health Care."

43. F. de Brantes and J. A. Camillus, "Evidence-Informed Case Rates: A New Health Care Payment Model" (New York: The Commonwealth Fund, April 2007).

44. F. de Brantes, M. B. Rosenthal, and M. Painter, "Building a Bridge from Fragmentation to Accountability—the Prometheus Payment Model," *New England Journal of Medicine* 361, no. 11 (2009): 1033–36.

45. Shih and others, "Organizing the U.S. Health Care Delivery System for High Performance."

46. S. Guterman, K. Davis, S. Schoenbaum, and A. Shih, "Using Medicare Payment Policy to Transform the Health System: A Framework for Improving Performance," *Health Affairs* Web exclusive (January 27, 2009), w238–w250, http://content.healthaffairs.org/cgi/content/full/28/2/w238?maxtoshow=&HITS=10&hits=10&RESULTFORMAT=&author1=guterman&andorexactfulltext=and&searchid=1&FIRSTINDEX=0&resourcetype=HWCIT.

CHAPTER FIVE

ACHIEVING THE VISION

Operational Challenges and Improvement

Bruce J. Genovese

Introduction

Collaboration among providers has long been felt to be at the core of any effort to improve efficiency and clinical performance of health care delivery in the United States.[1] Systemization of health care delivery has been lacking in many previous attempts to contain costs and improve care. Most efforts to align delivery system entities have occurred on a small scale and have involved only a portion of the hospitals and physicians in a geographic area. Despite evidence that they have a positive impact on cost and outcomes, integrated delivery models have not become the principal mode of health care delivery in the United States. A variety of barriers have prevented large-scale adoption of the integrated model.[2] Health care reform will ultimately be unsuccessful without a change in this dynamic.

This chapter discusses the operational value of and barriers to physician-hospital integration, collaboration, and alignment. The chapter also provides an example of a successful physician-hospital collaboration involving the Medicare Participating Heart Bypass Center Demonstration project.

Operational Value of Physician-Hospital Integration

The two principal agents of care delivery in the United States–physicians and hospitals—often work side by side, but not together. A more integrated approach to the continuum of care has the potential to improve outcomes, achieve cost effectiveness, and improve the satisfaction of both types of providers.[3] Simple improvements in the day-to-day operations of a hospital are the mechanisms through which these ends can be realized. Improved physician-hospital collaboration can result in a number of specific operational benefits, including, but not limited to, improved care coordination, improved availability of patient information, length-of-stay management, decreased duplication of diagnostic interventions, population-based prevention efforts, improved patient safety, improved responsiveness to external quality reporting requirements, economies of scale in the purchase of medical supplies and equipment, improved productivity, and improved after-hours specialty physician emergency room coverage. These opportunities are examined in the next section.

Improved Coordination of Care

Modern medicine is a good deal more complex than it used to be. Today, very few significant medical conditions are diagnosed and treated by only one physician. In fact, a physician caring for a patient in the hospital setting is almost always but one of several physicians attending that patient. Increasingly, a variety of other caregivers, often employed by the hospital, such as diagnostic technicians, clinical pharmacists, and physical therapists, are an integral part of the health care team.

However, the effectiveness of such a team can be quite dependent on the milieu in which it works. For example, in the care of a patient who has suffered a myocardial infarction, lifestyle counseling should begin while the patient is still in the hospital. But these lifestyle changes are not easy ones to adopt, especially if the need for change follows years of self-indulgence. To be effective, such cardiac rehabilitation should be a seamless and choate experience for the patient. This is most likely to occur if all the physicians and all the other caregivers, both in the hospital and later, are working off the same playbook. This coordination is most likely to occur in a setting where the physicians and hospital work in close alignment. This same principal applies to other significant and costly conditions such as stroke rehabilitation, serious wound care, chronic pulmonary disease, diabetes, and chronic mental illness.

Improved Availability of Patient Information

Another benefit of physician-hospital integration is the ability to efficiently share patient care information. An integrated electronic medical record, which is fully available both in the physician office and at the hospital, not only saves physician and patient time but enhances the effectiveness of patient care. For example, physicians are well aware that the accuracy of the medical history is markedly enhanced when previously obtained information—including diagnostic studies, procedures and operations, medications, allergies, and previous physical examination data—is always available, irrespective of the care setting. For one thing, such a system improves patient safety tremendously. For example, correlation of outpatient and inpatient medication records can result in the prevention of both in-hospital and postdischarge medication errors.

Another potential benefit of such information availability is a reduction in hospital readmission rates, particularly for patients with chronic conditions (for example, congestive heart failure, chronic pulmonary disease, and diabetes). Access to the full clinical story, as contained in the electronic medical record, can help guide decision making in the emergency department to help prevent an unnecessary readmission, such as for acute fluid overload in a patient with chronic congestive heart failure.

However, there are few settings today where such a seamless electronic medical record system exists, despite the fact that there are now many commercial vendors of such systems. They mostly exist in group-practice-based integrated delivery systems. It is there that the financial, cultural, and legal stars best align to support the installation and use of this tool.

Length-of-Stay Management

The advent of the Medicare diagnosis-related group (DRG) payment system and the use of this methodology by other payers created a conflict between attending physician and hospital financial incentives regarding inpatient length of stay (see Chapter Four). Physicians, who receive payment for each in-hospital patient encounter, do not have a financial incentive to prevent unnecessary hospital days. The hospital, in contrast, has an incentive to reduce expenses related to the length of stay in most instances, as revenue for the admission is fixed. However, cooperative efforts to reduce unnecessary length of stay can clearly lead to mutual benefits for patient, physician, and hospital, as has been demonstrated numerous times under shared-risk arrangements between physicians and hospitals related to managed care contracts. Such financial arrangements between physicians and hospitals can pass regulatory scrutiny only under certain circumstances (see Chapter Six). More widespread use of such arrangements will require new relationships between physicians and hospitals in many parts of the country.

This may already be happening. Many hospitals and some primary care physicians in independent practice have determined that inpatient care of patients can be more effectively provided by hospital-based internists (*hospitalists*), in terms of both appropriate length of stay and quality of care. Most such physicians are hospital employees, although in some settings, the hospitalist works for a hospital-affiliated medical group. Each model has its pros and cons. The hospitalist model itself has adherents and opponents. Nevertheless, this model of integration is quite common now and is on the rise.

Decreased Duplication of Diagnostic Tests

Fee-for-service payment can encourage the use of high-cost diagnostic studies by both physicians and hospitals. As a result, patients can be subject to redundant care processes (for example, diagnostic imaging) when seen by physicians in office-based practice, emergency room staff, hospitalists, and hospital-based specialists. Joint ownership of diagnostic testing equipment can serve to reduce unnecessary duplication of tests and resultant costs. In addition, in studies such as computerized tomography (CT) scanning, reduced redundancy can help patients avoid some of the potential long-term radiation-related complications of these procedures, including a higher risk of cancer. Single-photon emission computed tomography imaging, coronary computerized tomographic angiography, positron emission tomography scans, and cardiac magnetic resonance angiography studies all can be used to determine the presence of reduced blood flow to the heart muscle and the risk of heart attack. All are useful in certain situations. All are expensive. Rarely are all such tests required to be used in one individual. Yet uncoordinated care in an unintegrated delivery system can all too often lead to such a result.

Population-Based Preventive Care

Effective population-based preventive care requires a joint effort involving community hospitals, physicians, and government-sponsored public health agencies. Hospital organizations have the resources and community standing to support community events and educational efforts. However, many patients look to their personal physician for advice regarding preventive measures. Separate messages from these entities may conflict and thus result in confusion, as was seen in late 2009 during the H1N1 influenza pandemic. In addition, experience has shown that immunizations, including influenza immunizations, may be repeated needlessly because of lack of coordinated record keeping. Often this responsibility falls to the patient. Some are equipped for this duty. Others, because of lack of health literacy, dementia, or other causes, are not.

Joint prevention efforts will be more organized, more effective, and less costly in the setting of accountable care organizations working as one-stop-shopping partners with public health agencies. In turn, such organizations, especially those in risk-sharing payment relationships, will benefit from long-term reduced costs and improved outcomes, as will the population. The reduction of intensive care unit admissions and deaths due to seasonal influenza among the oldest elderly is a prime example of such a positive impact.

Improved Patient Safety

Improved patient safety in the hospital setting, as championed by the Institute for Healthcare Improvement, the Institute of Medicine, and the Joint Commission, among others, must be a cooperative effort between hospitals and the physicians who practice there. Currently, patient safety improvement initiatives are often carried out separately by hospital administrators and their medical staffs. These efforts would be more effective and broader reaching if a greater level of integration between physicians and hospitals existed. The resulting joint goals, appropriate incentives, and breakdown in organizational barriers could produce results in patient safety with remarkable speed and efficiency. For example, the operating room patient safety innovation known as the preoperative checklist requires involvement and support by the professional medical staff, the nursing staff, and the hospital administration to be consistently applied.[4] It often requires a difficult cultural realignment for surgeons and other physicians who may remain unconvinced of its value because the errors that the checklist seeks to prevent are rare and may occur only once or twice in the lifetime of a physician. This is where the administrative authority of a well-led group practice can have a major impact on the likelihood of such attitude adjustments becoming permanent.

Another benefit of coordination between physicians and hospitals in reducing preventable errors will be reduced professional and institutional medical liability costs. Improvements in the medical liability atmosphere of an institution can, in turn, reduce the practice of defensive medicine.

Improved Responsiveness to External Quality-Reporting Requirements

Both hospitals and physicians are under continued pressure by accrediting bodies and payers to report quality-related performance measures. Medicare, in particular, has established core measures which must be reported if hospitals are to receive full adjustments in payments annually. The Joint Commission and other accrediting bodies also develop criteria and targets to which hospitals must demonstrate compliance to receive accreditation, which is often required for participation in Medicare. Results of these efforts are (or will be) public and may influence patient and physician choice of institution. Physicians are also faced with future Medicare and other insurer requirements regarding quality measurement. The Medicare Physician Quality Reporting Initiative incentive program pays physicians for both the submission of a set of performance metrics and for e-prescribing. The successful fulfillment of these requirements and incentives can rely on cooperation between physicians and hospitals in some cases. Such cooperation is more likely to take place in an integrated setting where incentives for performance are aligned.

Economies of Scale in the Purchase of Supplies and Equipment

Hospitals face significant expenses related to the breadth of physician demands for specific supplies and equipment, such as orthopedic devices, cardiac and cardiac surgery interventional equipment, and electrophysiology devices (pacemakers and defibrillators). Many of these physician preferences are unrelated to quality and often are a consequence of habit or training experiences. They are not always fact-based preferences. Worse, on occasion, such preferences can represent a conflict-of-interest relationship with a particular producer or supplier. These individual requirements limit the hospital's ability to obtain volume purchasing discounts and long-term contracts. Further, the excess hospital purchasing costs resulting from low-volume purchases cannot be passed on to some payers, especially the Medicare program, because of DRG-based reimbursement.

The dynamic in an integrated delivery system can be quite different. The management structure of the physician group provides a platform for convening physicians in a particular specialty in order to identify, with the leadership of the hospital, specific supplies and equipment where the potential for cost savings exists. The specialists can then debate the merits of narrowing the range of these items to be purchased by the hospital, thus increasing the hospital's purchasing volume and its negotiating strength with suppliers. The physician group may be able to participate in the savings in certain situations.

Improved Productivity

Under the fee-for-service compensation system, lost work time results in a loss of income for both hospitals and physicians. For hospitals, inefficient use of fixed assets such as operating rooms has a negative impact on margins. For physicians, delays caused by waiting for operating rooms to be cleaned and turned around can lead to unproductive time in the locker room. The typical relationship between most physicians and hospitals is ill suited for improving institutional or professional productivity—such as by shortening operating room turnaround time—because of the complexity of standardizing work flows with large numbers of physicians in multiple specialties. But an integrated relationship between the parties with a shared incentive to promote more productive use of resources can result in faster transitions of this kind.

Specialty Physician Emergency Room Coverage

It is becoming increasingly difficult for hospitals to find after-hours on-call specialty coverage for their emergency rooms. This is primarily a consequence of the increased numbers of uninsured patients seeking such care, which increases bad debt for physician practices. This problem is also related to changing physician lifestyle preferences and the increase in two-career families where both spouses have child-care responsibilities, which makes leaving home at night difficult. Some hospitals have resorted to paying large nightly retainers to specialists simply to meet regulatory coverage requirements. Other hospitals are solving this problem either by hiring specialty physicians to work in the hospital on a full-time basis or establishing an integrated relationship with one or more group practices with after-hours emergency room coverage as a condition of the partnership. Again, this issue could be easily resolved in an integrated system.

Operational Barriers to Improved Integration

Given the potential benefits of physician-hospital integration described in the previous section, one might wonder why more progress has not been made in this direction. Some causes are intrinsic to the culture of physicians and hospitals, and some causes are extrinsic to these parties. Several examples of both are discussed in the following sections.

Difficulty of Forming Multispecialty Groups

Multispecialty group practice is key to improved efficiency and outcome improvement in clinical practice.[5] However, the disparity in income among different specialties can be a major deterrent to such integration. The way physician income is determined within a group can range from a simple salary-based model to a production and incentive-based model. Each model has its challenges and can be felt to be unfair by physicians. On the one hand, payment by salary provides a predictable income for physicians and promotes a sense of stability. However, a salary-based system requires that the group governance structure allocate income by specialty, a process which can lead to discord. In addition, salary-based groups require management processes to assure individual physician productivity. On the other hand, productivity-based payment can create quite large income disparities among specialties, often leading to either unhappiness among the lower-income physicians (such as primary care physicians) or disgruntlement among higher-paid specialists if the group decides to subsidize the income of the lower-paid physicians. Solving payment wars is critical to the ability to create and maintain a multispecialty group.

Beyond income issues, it can be difficult to establish a group culture, as described in Chapter Eight. Physicians are independent individuals, both by nature and training. Group practice requires a common infrastructure, which can mean that the environment in which a physician practices is not precisely what that physician would choose if fully independent. For example, the nursing staff is usually employed by the group, not by individual physicians. As a consequence, physicians may not like the nurse with whom they work. Not all physicians can manage such issues and be content. Others can. Thus, group practice is not for every physician.

In addition, independent practice physicians have generally been able to choose associates or partners with specific characteristics that they feel are important. As organizations become larger and more bureaucratic, colleagues become more diverse in personality, training, motivation, group orientation, and financial needs. That environment may not be tolerated by some physicians, who would hesitate to relinquish control over the choice of their associates. However, there is some reason to believe that this issue may be disappearing to some degree, as more Generation X and Y physicians, and especially women, join the practicing physician workforce. Interest in group practice appears to be higher in this newer cadre of physicians.

Nevertheless, the starting point for a successful physician-hospital integration effort is the establishment of a successful physician organization. At present, the rate of new multispecialty group formation lags behind the need.[6]

Lack of Payment Methodologies That Promote Group Formation

Some insurers offer managed care risk products through which physicians and hospitals can receive prospective payment for services. The Medicare Advantage program, as organized by some insurers, is an example of this model. Blue Cross of Massachusetts is currently experimenting with such forms of payment in the commercial sector as well.[7] Such payment models can create incentives for physicians and hospitals to collaborate. However, other insurers had unsatisfactory experiences with the capitation models in use in the 1990s and are not anxious to try this type of methodology again. Others frankly fear delivery system consolidation, because larger delivery system organizations can exercise more bargaining power in payment negotiations with insurers. Paradoxically, the experience of the 1990s did show that if payers do create payment methodologies that best benefit integrated organizations, then physicians and hospitals seem to be able to respond with movement toward structural integration. As part of health care reform, Congress has expressed an interest in the Medicare program studying the value of direct prospective payments to organized delivery systems (see Chapter Eleven).

Competition

There is growing competition between hospitals and physician groups, creating further impediments to integration. Many hospitals, particularly academic medical centers, support faculty practices that compete with community physicians. In addition, hospitals increasingly are recruiting physicians into salaried positions, particularly in primary care and obstetrics. This is sometimes because of a perceived community need, but generally to ensure an adequate referral network for the hospital's inpatient and outpatient services.

Increasingly, physicians and hospitals directly compete over outpatient diagnostic and therapeutic procedures. Physicians have added these functions to their own office practices to improve revenue, quality, and patient satisfaction. Because the bulk of the payment for many of these procedures is related to the technical (facility-related) component, rather than the professional component, this practice has proven very lucrative to physicians and physician groups. At the same time, the loss of such procedures has had a negative impact on hospital revenues and margins. In some communities, physicians have funded and built their own hospitals to compete with community hospitals, although Congress appears likely to soon curtail their ability to do this. In some areas of the country this competitive dynamic is so well established, and so much anger and distrust has been created between physician and hospitals, that efforts at integration have structural, financial, and human obstacles to overcome.

Different Business Cultures

As described in Chapter Eight, there are cultural differences between physicians and hospital leaders. The business model and culture of hospital organizations, particularly nonprofit entities, differs from the private practice model. The tendency for prolonged decision-making processes in what can be perceived as a very bureaucratic organization is contrary to the private practice culture. Many physicians share some common characteristics: a sense of self-direction, a conservative approach to government involvement in their business, a feeling of entitlement to a level of income and standard of living based on their stature and level of training, and an aversion to business lingo. A lack of business training, a for-profit mentality, and a need for prompt resolution of even complex problems are other characteristics of many physicians that make discussions with them regarding organization and collaboration difficult. These cultural differences make integration a difficult step for physicians to take.

Further, there is a serious gap in the financial education of physician leaders. Although many hospitals have developed physician leadership education opportunities, financial management training is not always part of this education. Independent consultants can facilitate negotiations involving physicians and hospitals, but physician leaders who understand the financial issues and can then educate their colleagues will have the most credibility and influence.

Compounding this issue is the lack of a business mentality in many physicians. Physicians have a different perspective regarding long-range planning, capital investments, financial reserves, strategic planning and goal setting, and the need to adjust to market conditions. As a result there has not been a tradition of understanding between physicians and hospital administrators, and this can inhibit integration efforts.

Physicians Disconnecting from Hospitals

Over the last several years there has been movement by both primary care physicians and specialists away from hospital-based activities. This trend has served to further separate, rather than integrate, physician-hospital activity. As discussed earlier, specialist physicians have developed free-standing diagnostic and surgical centers, in addition to performing procedures and testing in their offices that used to be performed in hospitals. In some cases, physician groups have built separate specialty hospitals, further disengaging from the community hospital setting.

Physicians have further disconnected with hospitals as the hospitalist movement has gained momentum. A significant percentage of primary care physicians no longer visit or *round on* their patients when they are admitted to the hospital. Hospitalists, some in independent hospital-based private practice and some employed or contracted by the hospital, often have full authority regarding the plan of care and the use of specialists. This can create a clinical gulf between the hospitalist and the outside physician, further alienating each from the other and breaking any psychological bond that could exist between the community-based physician and the hospital.

Lack of Consistent Quality Performance Measures

As described earlier, hospitals and physicians are required by payers (including Medicare), regulators (especially at the state level), and independent accrediting organizations (such as the Joint Commission and the National Committee for Quality Assurance) to provide information about the quality of care they deliver. Unfortunately, the measures required from physicians and from hospitals as part of these initiatives are often different, and so an opportunity can be missed to create incentives for physician-hospital collaboration on common goals. For example, Medicare has sponsored the creation of a voluntary quality-reporting program for physicians, known as the Physician Quality Reporting Initiative (PQRI), and a set of separate incentives for hospitals to improve patient safety and reduce unnecessary admissions. These and other initiatives have value because the process of quality measurement is complex and difficult and still in a formative stage. However, more attention should be given to measuring those kinds of activities that require close collaboration between hospitals and physicians and constructing rewards that are shared. To do so will not just improve quality but will help otherwise fractious parties find a set of mutual goals.

In the end, all providers—physicians and hospitals alike—want to be known for the delivery of high-quality care. Quality of care is their fundamental mission. And quality is the lingua franca that both hospitals and physicians can bring to the table in collaboration discussions. Without an increase in common goals in the area of quality measurement and reward, efforts to organize caregivers under the banner of patient care improvement will be less effective.

Different Information Systems

Physician-hospital integration efforts have been limited by the lack of a national standard for electronic health records and the resulting variability in products and systems that have been created or purchased by various hospital systems and physician groups. Often, systems have been acquired primarily to satisfy parochial requirements of each organization. Hospitals have adopted computerized provider order-entry technology to ensure accuracy and to track utilization. Some have implemented inpatient medical records.[8] Meanwhile, physician groups are purchasing electronic medical records that are compatible with their practice management systems and are fundamentally outpatient oriented.[9] At present, this lack of alignment in systems continues to be the rule, and it needs to be overcome to make physician-hospital integration easier technically. A national health care technology coordinator has been appointed in an effort to align health information technology. The goal of this office is to improve patient care and reduce excessive costs by enabling the exchange of information among providers.[10] Well-intentioned and expertly led as the federal efforts are, the task of establishing the correct standards to facilitate migration and linkage of these disparate legacy systems is complex and will take time.

Physician Inability to See Value in Integration

Finally, a significant barrier to improved physician-hospital integration is the simple fact that many physicians are not convinced there is sufficient value in integration. The vast majority of physicians feel they are currently providing good medical care and good service, with adequate access for patients. They are focused on individual patients and their outcomes. They see the work they do and the tests and procedures they perform as valuable and worth the expense to the patient and insurer. Rather than seeing value in integration, they see the potential for such a change to interfere with their patient relationships and their ability to provide the kind of customized care they feel they were trained to provide.

Physicians are aware of integrated delivery models, which are well known across the country. The Mayo Clinic, Kaiser Permanente, the Cleveland Clinic, the Henry Ford Health System, and others have been spoken of and written about widely. However, most physicians have not experienced firsthand the culture and patient care focus of these groups. This is in part related to the scattered location of these institutions. It is also related to the entrepreneurial spirit that prevented many newly trained physicians in the past from looking into positions in these settings. In addition, once in practice, most physicians have little contact with successful integrated groups. Less integrated models such as independent practice associations (IPAs) are available in many areas but don't give physicians the taste of what these major medical groups can provide.

Further, when considering a closer affiliation, hospitals and physicians often look back on negative experiences with integration as part of the growth of the managed care industry in the 1990s. This can be the case even if the individual hospitals and physicians were not directly involved in these failed experiments. Future efforts at physician-hospital integration will have to overcome some of the ill will and distrust that was often engendered during this period.

Operational Changes to Encourage Integration

Ultimately, the future of physician-hospital integration will be as much influenced by external forces as by the actions of physicians and hospital administrators. As well described in Chapter Six, there are a number of regulatory barriers to integration that will need to be addressed. Also critical will be efforts by payers, perhaps led by Medicare (see Chapter Four), to devise payment opportunities that provide incentives for integration. Standardization of electronic medical record technology will help. In addition, the development by payers and voluntary accrediting organizations of more performance measures that reflect outpatient-inpatient care coordination will be positive.

On the other hand, there are a set of actions that physicians and hospital administrators can take on their own to prepare the groundwork for future integration. An important step will be the evolution of more collaborative governance models, as described in Chapter Seven. In addition, collaboration on a number of important operational issues can be important first steps toward laying that groundwork.

As noted earlier, both hospitals and practicing physicians gain when the work flow processes in the hospital environment become more efficient. This is as true for the management of the emergency room, the patient floors, the laboratory and other hospital services as it is for the management of the operating room. A notable example of the benefits of this work is the multiyear project at the Virginia Mason Clinic in Seattle to adapt the lean production techniques of the Toyota automobile company to patient care activities at that hospital. Collaborative efforts between the physicians and hospital leaders at that integrated delivery system resulted in significant cost savings and allowed those reduced costs to be passed on to employers in the Seattle area, which was good for the reputation and the business stability of the entire enterprise. Those involved in this effort examined in extreme detail the work-flow processes throughout the hospital, making small and large changes to achieve their results.[11]

Another natural area for collaboration is quality and patient safety. The publication by the Institute of Medicine in 2000 of *To Err Is Human: Building a Safer Health System*, and the success of the work of Donald Berwick and his colleagues at the Institute for Healthcare Improvement (IHI) in reducing hospital medical errors have created a new focus on the safety of American hospitals.[12] Because most hospitals and their physicians share in the reputation or brand awareness of the institution, it is a matter of common interest that the hospital is perceived as safe for patients and that the institution scores well on measures of error prevention. Thus the avoidance of deep intravenous line infections, the reduction in postoperative pneumonias, and the prevention of decubitus ulcers (bedsores) in the elderly and infirm are to the benefit of physicians and the hospital, as well as patients. Each of these activities requires that the hospital have in place policies that describe the best practice for preventing the unwanted result. In some cases, specialized training is required for the nursing staff. In addition, the physicians need to be full participants in the activities, writing the correct orders and performing tasks as simple as thorough hand washing. Properly designed and executed, the results can be gratifying, and, as noted earlier, an initial collaborative success can begin to break down the barriers of mistrust between physicians and hospital administrators.

Ideally, in the wake of the 2009–2010 health care reform efforts, we are moving into a time when external forces and internal physician-hospital dynamics begin to better align. One prime example of such alignment could be implementation by the Medicare program of new payment alternatives for interested delivery systems. In anticipation of this set of activities, it may be helpful to examine one successful model of this from the recent past, the Medicare Participating Heart Bypass Center Demonstration, in which this author and his hospital participated.

Case Study: Saint Joseph Mercy Hospital

In 1988 in an effort to control the rapidly rising costs of coronary artery bypass graft surgery, the Health Care Financing Administration (HCFA, now the Centers for Medicare and Medicare Services) decided to determine the value of using bundled payments to physicians and hospitals as a partial solution to the problem (see Chapters One and Four). In response to a mail solicitation sent to 734 hospitals across the United States, 27 organizations submitted formal bids to be part of the proposed demonstration project. Four hospitals, including Saint Joseph Mercy Hospital (hereafter called St. Joseph's) in Ann Arbor, Michigan, were accepted into the program initially. St. Joseph's is a 550-bed, tertiary care, community teaching hospital that has provided high-level cardiac care since it opened in the early 1920s. The hospital at that time was a member of Mercy Health System (now Trinity Health) based in Farmington Hills, Michigan. Later, in 1993, three other hospitals were added.

The first four hospitals in the demonstration project began receiving bundled payments by June of 1991. Participating hospitals and physicians were allowed to divide the payment between them in any manner that they agreed upon. The demonstration lasted until the end of the second quarter of 1996, following which a formal evaluation was conducted for HCFA.[13]

In retrospect, the Medicare Participating Heart Bypass Center Demonstration experience at St. Joseph's was an example of a successful and mutually rewarding effort to join together primary care physicians and specialists using a bundled payment methodology. But that success was achieved only through the development of collaboration among previously disparate parties. At the inception of the Medicare demonstration, there were two competing cardiology groups, one cardiothoracic surgery group, and one vascular surgery group providing all the cardiovascular specialty care at the hospital. Single-specialty groups covered most other involved specialty areas, such as anesthesiology and pulmonology.

The demonstration project, as described earlier, provided a bundled payment to the participants for virtually all patient care services related to coronary artery bypass surgery with or without cardiac catheterization. Critical to the project was the mutual collaboration of the hospital, the cardiothoracic surgery group, and the two cardiology groups in designing the methodology for distribution of the revenue, as well as for negotiating the provision of other specialty services. The two competing cardiology groups had a history of cooperation in determining use of the cardiac catheterization laboratory, in the division of noninvasive study performance both in the outpatient and inpatient settings, and in sharing the on-call schedule. However, they were intensely competitive in both settings for referrals and consultations, the core of their business. The primary sources of income for the practices (consultation and invasive and noninvasive testing) were included in the demonstration project. As a result, both groups had to agree to participate in order for the project to be implemented. The rationale for the groups to participate included some expectation of increased volume related to publicity regarding the project and to improved revenue per case based on the negotiated division of the bundled payment. Other specialties such as pulmonology, vascular surgery, and infectious disease were included in the project through negotiated fixed-fee agreements.

Once the various stakeholders agreed to participate, they began efforts to improve the process of care and to reduce costs for the involved interventions. These efforts were facilitated by a consultant. Several major changes in the care processes were undertaken as a result of these discussions, including earlier postoperative extubation, earlier discharge from the intensive care unit, and earlier discharge (by almost two days) from the hospital. This improvement in efficiency ended up involving both Medicare and non-Medicare patients. Patients seemed to feel better more quickly and were on their feet sooner than had been the case previously. Cardiology input into the postoperative care of the patients was smoother than before, as there was not a need for formal consultation and billing processes.

The project resulted in a closer working relationship between the cardiology groups as well as between cardiology and cardiothoracic surgery. During the course of the project the two cardiology groups began merger discussions and eventually joined to form one group. Discussions with the hospital led to a closer relationship between the involved physician groups and the hospital administration, as well as increased physician awareness of the tangible benefits of cost efficiency. The resulting collaboration might have been extended to other patient care interventions if Medicare had decided to broaden the demonstration project. Across the four participating hospitals the demonstration project saved Medicare $17 million in 27 months. At St. Joseph's, the project increased the hospital's margin for coronary artery bypass surgery with cardiac catheterization by 62 percent.[14] The Health Care Financing Administration followed quality data for the participating hospitals carefully and showed stable to improving quality over the course of the demonstration.

At St. Joseph's, the project clearly demonstrated the potential for the bundled payment methodology to lead toward collaboration among physician groups and hospital organizations while promoting improved care and cost efficiencies. However, the demonstration was not expanded. In fact it was discontinued at the end of the study period. Reportedly HCFA's plans to expand the project were curtailed by budgetary issues at the agency.[15]

St. Joseph's returned to fee-for-service reimbursement for bypass surgery. However, the benefits of the project related to patient care persisted, including shorter lengths of stay, improved early postoperative status, and improved functional capacity at discharge from the hospital. In addition, the project fostered a closer working relationship between cardiologists and surgeons, as well as between physicians and the hospital, which persists to this day.

Conclusion

The lack of *systemness* in U.S. health care delivery is largely responsible for the relatively higher cost of health care in the United States and perhaps contributes to lower quality as well. The prevalence of the differing business models found in physician groups and in hospital organizations, competition between the two, and most important, the nature of the payment system are largely responsible for this situation.

Physician integration is necessary for improving the systemness of health care delivery. Although there has been growth in single-specialty groups in recent years, multispecialty physician organizations have been slower to develop, in part because of interspecialty competition for patients and revenue. Payment incentives designed to foster a more collaborative approach across specialties would not only result in better coordination of patient care but would also likely improve cost containment. Examples such as the Mayo Clinic and Kaiser Permanente have demonstrated the positive affects of multispecialty collaboration over many decades of existence.

Incentives to create physician-hospital integration are also needed. The major barriers to hospital and physician integration relate to financial and control issues. Aligning incentives for hospitals and physicians will involve cultural adjustments for these entities. The ability to compromise regarding decision-making processes and investment priorities is vital. The experience at St. Joseph's with the Medicare demonstration project showed two things. First, it showed the impact of payment incentives on the willingness of disparate parties within the hospital environment to put aside differences and work collaboratively. Second, it showed that such collaboration can have salutary and lasting effects. It is time for the Medicare program to begin to lead such advances again.

Notes

1. W. A. Pestasnick, "Hospital-Physician Relationships: Imperative for Clinical Enterprise Collaboration," *Frontiers of Health Service Management* 24, no. 1 (2009): 3–10.
2. M. Taylor, "Working Through the Frustrations of Clinical Integration," *Hospital Health Network* 82, no. 1 (2008): 34–37.
3. R. A. Berenson, P. A. Ginsburg, and J. H. May, "Hospital-Physician Relations: Cooperation, Competition, or Separation?" *Health Affairs* Web exclusive (December 5, 2006), w31–w43, http://content.healthaffairs.org/cgi/reprint/26/1/w31.
4. A. B. Haynes and others, "A Surgical Safety Checklist to Reduce Morbidity and Mortality in a Global Population," *New England Journal of Medicine* 360, no. 5 (2009): 491–99.
5. S. M. Shortell and L. Casalino, "Accountable Care Systems for Comprehensive Healthcare Reform" (paper for the workshop "Organization and Delivery of Care and Payment to Providers," Center for Advanced Study in the Behavioral Sciences, Stanford University, CA, March 1–2, 2007), http://freshthinking.org/docs/workshop_070301/ShortellCasalinoDeliverySystemModelsRevise9.pdf.
6. H. H. Pham and P. B. Ginsburg, "Unhealthy Trends: The Future of Physician Services," *Health Affairs* 26, no. 6 (2007): 1586–98.
7. R. Steinbrook, "The End of Fee-for-Service Medicine? Proposals for Payment Reform in Massachusetts," *New England Journal of Medicine* 361, no. 11 (2009): 1036–38.
8. A. K. Jha and others, "Use of Electronic Records in U.S. Hospitals," *New England Journal of Medicine* 360, no. 16 (2009): 1628–37.
9. C. M. DesRoches and others, "Electronic Health Records in Ambulatory Care: A National Survey of Physicians," *New England Journal of Medicine* 359, no. 1 (2008): 50–60.
10. U.S. Department of Health and Human Services, "HHS Names David Blumenthal as National Coordinator for Health Information Technology" (press release), March 20, 2009, http://www.hhs.gov/news/press/2009pres/03/20090320b.html (accessed December 18, 2009).
11. G. Kaplan, "Testimony Before the Medicare Payment Advisory Committee," Washington, D.C., September 7, 2006, http://www.medpac.gov (accessed November 10, 2009).
12. Institute of Medicine, *To Err Is Human: Building a Safer Health System* (Washington, D.C.: National Academies Press, 2000); J. Whittington, T. Simmonds, and D. Jacobsen, "Reducing Hospital Mortality Rates (Part 2)," IHI Innovation Series White Paper, 2005, http://www.ihi.org/IHI/Results/WhitePapers/ReducingHospitalMortalityRatesPart2.htm (*must be a member of IHI Web site to access this file*).
13. J. Cromwell and others, "Medicare Participating Heart Bypass Center Demonstration: Executive Summary—Final Report" (Waltham, MA: Health Economics Research, July 24, 1998).
14. Cromwell and others, "Medicare Participating Heart Bypass Center Demonstration."
15. R. Coulam, R. Feldman, and B. Dowd, "Don't Forget to Save Medicare: Competitive Pricing, Not Price Controls" (Washington, D.C.: American Enterprise Institute for Public Policy Research, July 17, 2009), 1.

CHAPTER SIX

OVERCOMING BARRIERS TO IMPROVED COLLABORATION AND ALIGNMENT

Legal and Regulatory Issues

Robert F. Leibenluft
William M. Sage

Introduction

Contractual, financial, and structural relations between physicians and hospitals in the United States are heavily influenced by law. No matter how laudable the goal, any dramatic change in those arrangements in connection with national health reform will encounter an array of legal barriers with different histories and rationales. Some are imposed by federal law, some by state law. Unsurprisingly, many are the direct or indirect result of the enactment of Medicare and Medicaid in the 1960s—America's most serious attempt thus far to assure medical care to its citizens—which dramatically altered public investment in the health care system and public expectations regarding its performance.

For the purpose of examining the legal barriers that might become important in the near future, this chapter posits a change from the currently fragmented system of health care delivery to a less fragmented system. The chapter assumes that one key element of that change is replacing payment policies that emphasize fees for individual services with policies that encompass complete episodes of care or sustained periods of medical need. It assumes as well that defragmentation of health care delivery requires shifting from an information-poor environment to an environment where much more is known and shared about the price and quality of health care, both among providers and with patients, purchasers, and the public.

Even in the heat of debate over a major health reform law, it is not clear exactly how these changes might occur. Based on widespread public distrust of what has come to be called managed care, change is unlikely to be led by private insurance organizations seeking rewards in the marketplace. But neither is it likely to be engineered by a rapid overhaul of government purchasing, whether through Medicare, Medicaid, or a so-called public option. Rather, a mixed model of health reform is to be expected, making it necessary to address related legal issues in the context of transitions as well as desirable long-term outcomes. Ideally, the legal and policy environment can be designed in the form of a ratchet, promoting complementary changes in payment methods, information reporting, and the cooperative structure of provider organizations while preventing the system from sliding back into disarray.

This chapter assumes that legal change is necessary but not sufficient for health system change. If powerful new payment policies and informational transparency initiatives fail to materialize, no amount of legal maneuvering will matter. However, because law is a pervasive feature of the American health care system, legal change is likely necessary for other changes to occur. Legal change is also a key consideration in the politics of health care reform, because legal issues that are not under the direct control of a reforming body (such as state laws that Congress is unable or unwilling to address) are often cited by opponents as reasons why reform should not proceed.

The laws affecting physician-hospital relationships that are discussed in this chapter are based on a small number of identifiable theories of the public interest in health care. One category of laws, including the antitrust laws, is motivated by concern over impediments to effective competition in health care as an industry. A second category, notably fraud and abuse laws, is motivated by the risks of financial exploitation associated with provider payment mechanisms. A third category, exemplified by the laws of tax exemption, is motivated by public desire to support socially beneficial activities. A fourth, rather broad category responds to patient vulnerability by attempting to ensure quality and professionalism (through, for example, licensing and medical malpractice laws).

The chapter begins by examining the three core federal issues of antitrust, fraud and abuse, and tax exemption.[1] It next discusses major state legal regimes that influence the structure of physician-hospital relationships: professional licensing, medical staff credentialing, corporate practice of medicine, insurance, and medical malpractice.[2] The chapter ends with the authors' assessment of the top priority areas for legal reform to promote delivery system reform.

Antitrust

Antitrust law differs from the other issues considered in this chapter because it is a general law to which the health care system has increasingly become subject, whereas the rest are specialized laws enacted specifically for application to health care. The two main federal antitrust statutes, the Sherman Act and the Clayton Act, were enacted in 1890 and 1914, respectively, but were not initially applied to professional activities. In the mid-twentieth century, antitrust law began to be invoked to prevent joint exclusionary behavior by organized physicians against rival health professionals (for example, chiropractors) and physicians who accepted unconventional commercial terms (for example, prepaid group practices). Medicine had become so economically powerful that, if allowed to exercise more self-regulatory authority than the generous amount already granted it by law, it could destroy erstwhile competitors rather than accommodate and absorb them (as it had done with homeopaths and osteopaths). In the 1970s and 1980s, moreover, public reaction against professions and other paternalistic elites led to a series of Supreme Court decisions holding them subject to essentially the same rules of competition as commercial ventures. Leading cases involved law (*Goldfarb*), engineering (*Society of Professional Engineers*), and dentistry (*Indiana Federation of Dentists*) but are as applicable to medicine as the cases involving physicians (*Maricopa County Medical Society, Jefferson Parish Hospital District*).[3]

Today the health care industry accounts for a surprisingly large amount of antitrust litigation, particularly private lawsuits by physicians against other physicians and hospitals.[4] The extent of medical antitrust litigation derives in large part from the massive injection of funds provided by health insurance, especially Medicare. Federal antitrust enforcement often involves surprisingly small communities, with major merger litigation occurring in towns such as Grand Rapids, Michigan; Poplar Bluff, Missouri; and Evanston, Illinois.[5] With sufficient capital, even modest geographic markets became profitable enough to maintain competition among hospitals and specialists. Additionally, private antitrust suits often arose from alterations of traditional medical staff relationships as the result of Medicare's adoption of prospective payment for hospitals in 1982, followed in the next decade by selective contracting with managed care organizations (see Chapter Four).

The quest for greater clinical efficiency continues to challenge courts to distinguish competitive collaboration from anticompetitive collusion, especially as fragmented delivery systems begin to consolidate and integrate. Government antitrust enforcement typically involves efforts by otherwise independent and competing providers to collectively negotiate payment rates with private health plans. In contrast, collective attempts by providers to secure higher government reimbursement are generally shielded from antitrust challenge as protected First Amendment activity under the so-called Noerr-Pennington doctrine.[6]

Antitrust law is often described as a possible obstacle to greater physician-hospital collaboration. However, many collaborations are unlikely to raise significant antitrust issues, generally because they do not involve competing entities or do not relate to price or other competitively sensitive issues. Collaborations that involve agreements among independent providers who compete—or potentially compete—with each other, and that relate to negotiations with health plans, can raise more difficult antitrust questions, but in many cases these may not be insurmountable.

Although the antitrust enforcers have provided some useful guidance in this area, more could be done to help providers grappling with health reform distinguish between circumstances under which joint efforts raise legal concerns and those in which there is little antitrust risk. Over the longer term, moreover, different antitrust issues may arise if physician-hospital collaborations such as accountable care organizations (ACOs) become so successful that they bestow market power on the participating providers and impede effective local competition.

Federal antitrust laws apply to all sectors of the economy, including health care providers. The three principal federal antitrust statutes are aimed at (1) agreements between independent economic entities that unreasonably restrain trade (Sherman Act § 1), (2) predatory or exclusionary conduct to obtain or maintain a monopoly (Sherman Act § 2), and (3) mergers or acquisitions that threaten to substantially lessen competition (Clayton Act § 7).

The goal of these laws is to promote competition, which is assumed to bring lower prices, increased quality, and innovation. There are of course a number of reasons why health care markets may depart from classic economic competitive models, including third-party payment, the role of employers as insurance purchasing agents, extensive regulation, the lack of reliable information about quality, the asymmetry of information between providers and patients, the existence of large government payers, the need to provide health services to the uninsured, and the involvement of nonprofits and professionals who may be guided by norms other than profit maximization. Nevertheless, the current health care system is based on a competitive model, and arrangements among providers that implicate the antitrust laws will be subject to attack by both government antitrust enforcers and private litigants seeking treble damages.

Agreements in Restraint of Trade: Sherman Act § 1

Currently, the most common type of antitrust issues raised by physician-hospital collaboration concern Sherman Act §1, when such collaboration involves agreements among independent and otherwise competing physicians.

In certain circumstances, physician-hospital collaborations raise issues under the antimonopolization provisions of Sherman Act § 2. This might occur, for example, where a dominant hospital locks up its physician staff so they cannot create freestanding competitive ventures or work at other hospitals. Collaborations that involve the merger of competing physician practices could raise issues under Clayton Act § 7. However, at least currently, these situations are relatively rare, compared to the much more common antitrust issues that arise under Sherman Act § 1.

Sherman Act § 1 is both broad and simple—it prohibits "[e]very contract, combination . . . or conspiracy, in restraint of trade."[7] Because virtually every contract can restrain trade in some respects, the statute has been interpreted to ban only unreasonable restraints of trade—that is, where the anticompetitive effects outweigh any likely procompetitive benefits. A finding that an agreement is anticompetitive requires evidence of actual anticompetitive effects or a showing that the parties to the agreement had market power in a properly defined product and geographic market. This is a difficult burden to bear; as a result, conduct that is evaluated under this so-called rule of reason is typically very difficult to challenge successfully.

However, in decisions spanning more than a century, courts have identified certain agreements that are viewed as so likely to have an anticompetitive effect that they can be condemned without any inquiry into the relevant markets that might be affected by the agreement. Such agreements are per se unlawful, and the parties are not given an opportunity to defend their conduct by claiming that their prices are reasonable or that their conduct is procompetitive. Examples of per se illegal conduct include price-fixing and geographic or product market allocation agreements among competitors.

A crucial issue in any physician-hospital collaboration, therefore, is whether the relevant agreements will be summarily condemned as per se illegal or whether they should be evaluated under the rule of reason. According to the *Antitrust Guidelines for Collaborations Among Competitors* of the U.S. Department of Justice and the Federal Trade Commission, the latter is warranted where otherwise competing entities join together in an "efficiency-enhancing integration of economic activity" and "enter into an agreement that is reasonably related to the integration and reasonably necessary to achieve its pro-competitive benefits."[8] One way to appreciate the distinction between per se and rule of reason cases is to consider mergers among competing firms, which necessarily will result in formerly competing entities jointly setting prices. Such mergers are not condemned outright because it is assumed that the merged firm will have both the ability and the incentive to integrate its operations and thereby achieve efficiencies. Accordingly, the merger is reviewed under a rule of reason analysis that considers market concentration and other factors to determine whether any loss in competition is likely to outweigh possible efficiencies that could be achieved only through the merger.

With joint agreements that fall short of a full merger—as is often the case in physician-hospital collaborations—the likelihood that the parties will engage in efficiency-enhancing integration cannot be assumed, and a rule of reason analysis is not guaranteed. Even if an arrangement includes more than just an agreement on prices, the question remains whether the pricing agreement is really necessary or whether the efficiencies likely could be achieved in a manner involving less restrictive alternatives.

Antitrust Analysis of Provider Collaborations

An antitrust analysis of a given collaboration among health care providers involves four questions, which are diagrammed in Figure 6.1:

1. **Does the collaboration involve agreements that might be construed as per se illegal?** If the collaboration does not involve an agreement among competitors relating to the prices they will charge, the customers they will serve, or other matters that arguably could be condemned as per se illegal, then the initiative will be analyzed under the rule of reason. Although this does not mean there are no potential antitrust concerns, the antitrust risks are much less serious, as a challenge will depend on the ability of a complainant to demonstrate that the parties have market power and that their conduct, on balance, will have an anticompetitive effect.

2. **Is there sufficient integration to avoid per se condemnation so that the joint venture can be analyzed under the rule of reason; that is, does the venture have the potential to achieve substantial efficiencies?** Assuming that the venture does involve agreements that, standing alone, might be per se illegal, the next question is whether such agreements are naked restraints or are related to what the federal antitrust agencies have called "an efficiency-enhancing integration of economic activity" short of an actual merger into a single legal entity.

3. **Even if there is substantial integration, are the competitive restraints ancillary to the venture's procompetitive goals?** If a collaboration involves substantial integration, the next step is to examine the agreements made in connection with the joint venture to determine whether they are ancillary, that is, related and reasonably necessary to achieve the procompetitive goals of the venture.

4. **Will the joint venture, on balance, have anticompetitive effects?** If the competitive restraints are ancillary to the joint venture's procompetitive

FIGURE 6.1   SHERMAN ACT § 1 ANALYSIS

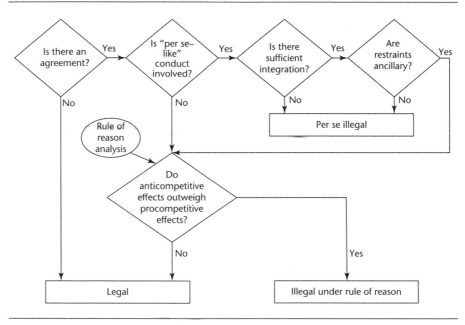

Source: Authors' analysis.

goals, then it is necessary to determine under the rule of reason whether, on balance, the venture will be anticompetitive. This assessment involves two steps: a further examination of the nature of the relevant agreements and the type of competitive harm and benefits that may result; and an assessment of competitive conditions in the market, including whether the parties to the joint venture will have market power.

For physician-hospital collaborations that involve agreements among competitors relating to the prices they will charge or the customers they will serve, the first issue is to determine whether there is sufficient clinical or financial integration between the parties to avoid per se condemnation. The 1996 *Statements of Antitrust Enforcement Policy in Health Care* (hereinafter *Health Care Policy Statements*) from the U.S. Department of Justice (DOJ) and Federal Trade Commission (FTC) focus on whether a collaboration between providers involves such integration. Guidance from the antitrust agencies is fairly straightforward with respect to how financial integration might be demonstrated. Financial integration exists where providers provide services at a shared capitated rate or where payment is subject to a substantial financial withhold depending on whether group performance goals are met. Financial integration may also be present where physicians in different specialties collaborate to provide complementary services for a complex or extended course of treatment and agree to accept a fixed predetermined payment for the entire episode of care (see Chapter Four for more on such episode-based payment strategies). In such arrangements, a failure to achieve collective goals across the venture results in lost revenue for all participants; as a result, the collaborators have strong incentives to achieve efficiencies that they would be unlikely to accomplish on their own.

Although capitation and withholds can provide assurance to hospitals and physicians that their collaborative activities will fall safely outside the per se box, both providers and payers have been less willing to enter into these types of contracts in recent years. Accordingly, the arrangements may need to rely on some form of clinical integration. Unfortunately, guidance from the federal antitrust enforcers as to what constitutes clinical integration is much less specific than the guidance on financial integration. Among other things, the antitrust agencies worry that their approval of certain arrangements in health care might be used to inappropriately justify arrangements in other industries or contexts. More fundamentally, reluctance to clearly define clinical integration may be due to how the FTC and DOJ view their roles, which is as enforcement officials—not as regulators. The statutes they enforce, unlike many other statutes that apply to health care entities, are written very broadly and apply to all industry sectors. The agencies realize that they lack the expertise and resources to promulgate regulations that could possibly address all kinds of health care collaborative efforts, and that attempts to be prescriptive about the details of market structure or conduct would inevitably deter innovation.

In the *Health Care Policy Statements*, the agencies state that clinical integration programs typically involve (1) mechanisms to monitor and control health care utilization to control costs and assure quality; (2) selectively choosing participating providers; and (3) significant investment of capital, both financial and human, in the necessary infrastructure.

Private parties can seek advisory opinions from the FTC or DOJ before they embark on particular initiatives, but such efforts are expensive and time consuming and are limited by their terms to the specific arrangement for which an opinion is sought. Moreover, because the agencies lack the ability to do a full-scale investigation and are reluctant to establish precedents that may be used in future unforeseen contexts, the opinions tend to be very conservative. In four advisory opinions involving real-world clinical integration initiatives, the FTC has examined specific proposals and provided more insight into why three such proposals should be allowed to proceed without challenge by the agency, and in one case explained why the proposal was problematic.[9]

In 2007 the American Hospital Association (AHA), in an effort to provide more extensive guidance to its member hospitals and other providers, released its *Guidance for Clinical Integration*.[10] The document addresses practical considerations in developing a clinical integration program and also expands on the legal analysis provided in the *Health Care Policy Statements* and FTC advisory opinions.

If a proposed physician-hospital collaboration includes sufficient integration to avoid per se condemnation, the next step in an antitrust analysis is to determine whether the competitive restraints are ancillary (in other words, incidental but necessary) to the venture's procompetitive goals. Consider two hospitals that form a joint venture to buy a mobile lithotripsy unit to provide services half of the time at each of the hospitals. Agreements regarding the purchase, operation, and sale of the technical component of the lithotripsy services (including the price for such services) are likely to be viewed as ancillary to the joint venture. However, an agreement regarding the prices for services not furnished through the joint venture (for example, the daily hospital room charge) is likely to be viewed as not ancillary to the joint venture, and will be condemned as per se illegal. Thus, this step of the analysis requires consideration of the subjects of any agreements the parties make, to ensure that they are related and reasonably necessary to achieving the legitimate goals of the joint venture.[11] In the context of provider clinical integration efforts, the antitrust enforcers emphasize that even if a collaboration is well considered and has lofty goals, it still must explain why joint negotiations with health plans are reasonably necessary to achieve these objectives.[12]

In sum, few physician-hospital collaborations will raise significant antitrust issues. If the initiatives do not involve joint negotiations by competitors with health plans, restrict the ability of the participants to make arrangements with other providers or health plans, or otherwise involve competitively sensitive issues, the arrangements will be assessed under the rule of reason, and in most circumstances, will not be subject to serious scrutiny.

Implications of Antitrust Law for ACOs

As noted, physician-hospital collaboration should raise few antitrust issues if the collaboration does not involve joint negotiation by competing independent providers about the fees they receive from health plans. Collaborations to improve quality or to more effectively deliver services under an administered price set by Medicare should not raise serious antitrust risks either. Collaborations that do involve joint negotiations with health plans will face more antitrust scrutiny, but generally they should be able to survive review as long as they reflect substantial clinical integration and as long as joint negotiations with payers are integral to the venture's legitimate goals.

Arrangements whereby providers agree to furnish services for an episode of care for a predetermined fee, provided that they lack market power, should pass antitrust scrutiny because of the financial integration that exists. However, even an appropriately integrated physician-hospital collaboration—such as the ACO models presented in Chapter Three—could be subject to antitrust challenge if it confers local market power on the participants. This could occur, for example, if a collaboration includes a very large percentage of the physicians in a community, particularly if the physicians are exclusive participants who will not contract with health plans outside the collaboration agreement. Alternatively, a collaboration between a dominant hospital provider and a large percentage of its medical staff may raise concerns about increasing further the hospital's market power or about making entry or expansion by competing hospitals or freestanding providers more difficult. Such scenarios will involve a balancing of the potential procompetitive and anticompetitive effects under antitrust law's rule of reason— an expensive, prolonged, and potentially difficult exercise. By and large, however, these will be issues for the future—arising only when ACOs have thrived and are threatening to become dominant. Unless hospitals and physicians are joining forces for the purpose of opposing innovation, antitrust law should not represent a barrier to the creation of collaborative arrangements where few currently exist.

In the short term, the biggest challenge for policymakers and antitrust enforcers will be to ensure that providers have sufficient guidance and that they understand that antitrust should not stand in the way of legitimate collaborative endeavors. Because antitrust analysis is so fact specific, there is no bright line that can be drawn between what is lawful and what is not. Antitrust enforcers are unlikely to establish very specific rules for collaborations, and indeed, such efforts would be counterproductive if they were too restrictive and locked providers into a limited set of market relationships. Still, the antitrust agencies could do more to emphasize that they are receptive to genuine efforts by collaborating hospitals and physicians to improve the care provided. They could also do a better job of explaining antitrust principles, so that providers can understand whether or not their efforts will prompt close antitrust scrutiny.

Fraud and Abuse

Laws falling under the rubric of fraud and abuse are almost always directed at undesirable financial practices, as opposed to clinical ones, although a half-hearted effort was made during the 1990s to use false claims statutes to police quality-related misrepresentations by health plans. Health care fraud and abuse laws exist at both state and federal levels and may apply to either publicly or privately financed care. The best-known such laws are federal criminal statutes and related civil provisions enforced by the Office of the Inspector General (OIG) of the U.S. Department of Health and Human Services (HHS). These statutes are intended to prevent abuses of federal health programs, mainly Medicare and Medicaid. Because punishing bad actors appeals more broadly across the political spectrum than does systematic restructuring of the health care system, the scope and severity of fraud and abuse laws have increased steadily with the growth of government health expenditures since Medicare was enacted in 1965.

Differences between antitrust law and fraud law highlight the pervasiveness of market distortions in health care. These two major sources of structural oversight for health care delivery converge only in privileging unilateral conduct by single entities receiving direct payment, which is not a realistic solution to rampant, unproductive fragmentation in the U.S. health care system. Otherwise, the two legal regimes diverge in both goals and means. As discussed earlier, antitrust law readily allows reasonable contractual arrangements in the production of goods and services, condemning only (1) situations in which the combining entities have sufficient power to raise prices with impunity and (2) naked restraints of trade (for example, price-fixing or division of markets) that cannot possibly benefit consumers. In particular, antitrust law seldom prohibits vertical agreements along the chain of production, reasoning that these relationships are likely to improve efficiency and seldom raise the risk of bottlenecking inherent in horizontal agreements among competitors at a single point (such as manufacturers of a finished product). Moreover, because aggressive behavior among competitors is generally preferable to passivity, antitrust law examines the competitive effects of market conduct, not its motivation.

In contrast, health care fraud laws assume that some providers and suppliers will impermissibly manipulate payment practices to receive larger amounts than those to which they are entitled. This assumption is based on several historical aspects of health care payment: administered rather than competitive pricing; payment by third parties rather than by the individual receiving services; physicians' virtually unfettered professional discretion to make referrals and issue orders for additional diagnosis and treatment; and lack of measurable outcomes associated with those services. Fragmentation of health care delivery worsens these risks by presenting countless opportunities for quid pro quo agreements among providers who perform different tasks. As a result, vertical agreements are more closely scrutinized under fraud and abuse laws than horizontal agreements, foreclosing many contractual arrangements that would almost certainly be procompetitive (and thus raise no antitrust concerns) in a less regulated industry.

In addition, criminal law is at the core of fraud enforcement, making unlawful intent rather than ill effect a constitutionally required element of successful prosecutions. Because of this touchstone, fraud law lacks a general economic construct such as market power to distinguish harmful from harmless activities, and relies instead on complex regulatory exceptions and safe harbors that seldom keep pace with ongoing changes in the industry. This is especially true of federal civil prohibitions against physician self-referral (Stark laws), which were enacted as strict liability offenses in order to spare the government the burden of proving unlawful intent but which therefore must be specified in excruciating detail in statute or regulations.

Consider the plight of providers who rely on financial or clinical integration to survive antitrust scrutiny of their joint negotiations with private payers. To establish the kind of integration needed to avoid per se condemnation, otherwise independent physicians may subject themselves to financial incentives that might improve quality or reduce unnecessary care. Alternatively, a hospital may wish to contribute information technology infrastructure and staff resources to assist physicians' joint clinical activities. Such incentives and contributions, however procompetitive from an antitrust perspective, can violate antikickback, self-referral, and civil monetary penalty provisions, as well as the federal tax exemption laws discussed later in this chapter.

The following section describes the four major federal fraud and abuse prohibitions: the antikickback statute, the self-referral (Stark) laws, the civil false claims act, and restrictions on paying physicians to withhold necessary services from patients. For each law, we discuss its historical and conceptual underpinnings as well as its implications for physician-hospital collaboration.

Kickbacks

As noted in Chapters Two and Four, Medicare's structural inability to contain costs was apparent shortly after its enactment in 1965: physicians were promised customary and prevailing fees; hospital and physician claims were paid separately by "Blues" plans acting as fiscal intermediaries and carriers but using public funds instead of their own; and the government had pledged noninterference in medical practice. By 1972, medical inflation was sufficiently worrisome to prompt Congress to amend Medicare to adopt, among other things, a prohibition on kickbacks, bribes, and rebates.[13] In the decades that followed, this rule was expanded to create a sweeping criminal indictment of any remuneration solicited or received by any person that was intended, even in part, to induce a Medicare or Medicaid referral.[14] Consequently, most contractual arrangements between manufacturers of medical products and service providers or between two different types of service provider present at least a theoretical risk of federal prosecution.

Many payments or services that hospitals might reasonably offer admitting physicians to promote loyalty and preserve patient flow—and therefore improve physician-hospital alignment—also constitute illegal remuneration. Examples include income guarantees, low-cost office space, and malpractice coverage. For this reason, the antikickback statute has emerged as a serious obstacle to gainsharing (shared savings) programs in which hospitals and physicians collaborate to improve efficiency of care for admitted patients and divide the associated financial savings (see Chapter Four). At present, the only gainsharing programs spared the risk of fraud enforcement are those being conducted directly under the auspices of the Centers for Medicare and Medicaid Services (CMS) as demonstration projects.[15]

The OIG periodically issues detailed regulations describing specific practices that it will refrain from prosecuting (safe harbors) and will respond to formal requests for advisory opinions, but these are troubling for two reasons. First, the government often must narrowly define practice matters best left to private innovation, such as when ancillary services are in a physician's office or what factors may or may not be considered in establishing the fair market value of contractual obligations. Second, the government cannot read the minds of providers regarding their intent to induce or reward referrals and therefore must frame advisory opinions around likely effects of the proposed conduct even though the antikickback statute focuses on unlawful purpose.

Physician Self-Referral

It is often said that the most expensive medical technology is a physician's pen. Roughly two-thirds of health care costs are incurred as the result of a physician's orders, largely funded by third parties rather than patients themselves. Beginning in the 1970s and 1980s, entrepreneurs exploited physicians' financial influence by offering them incentives of various kinds to supplement their income by referring patients to particular suppliers. For example, several ventures sold passive ownership interests in clinical laboratories to physicians who were in a position to send patients for testing at the owned facilities. Although physician financing of ancillary medical services was an established practice in small communities that might not otherwise be able to raise the necessary capital, the newer arrangements proliferated in Florida and other populous states with a high density of Medicare beneficiaries, and they seemed designed more to bilk the federal government than to increase access or service quality.

Curtailing abuse of this sort became a personal crusade for House Ways and Means Health Subcommittee Chairman Fortney (Pete) Stark of California. Congress enacted its first prohibition on physician self-referral to clinical laboratories (known as Stark I) in 1989 and followed that legislation with a broader ban (Stark II) in 1993.[16] The Stark laws respond to evidence that both legitimate suppliers and opportunistic financial promoters were encouraging physicians to invest in joint professional-commercial ventures to induce referrals at higher prices and in higher volumes than would be the case for arm's-length transactions. The more medical technology was developed in the 1980s and 1990s, and the more downward pressure was placed on fees for basic services such as office visits, the more attractive such schemes became as a source of supplemental income for physicians.

Although the Stark laws apply only to physicians and only to certain designated health services, they subject violators to strict liability, regardless of intent, and impose serious (though not criminal) penalties. Accordingly, a wide range of financial relationships between physicians and hospitals—whether ownership, investment, or compensation arrangements—that might serve to coordinate care are precluded for no reason other than that the physicians refer patients for inpatient or outpatient services at the hospitals. To be allowed, conduct needs to fall within an explicit, highly detailed statutory or regulatory exception. For example, hospitals and physicians cannot joint venture specialized services such as invasive cardiology for which the hospital will bill Medicare, even if the joint venture is cost effective. At the same time, questionably efficient structures generate excessive enthusiasm because they happen to be permissible. Physician-owned specialty hospitals, for example, have proliferated because a Stark exception allows physicians to invest in "whole hospitals" but not in particular clinical departments in a general hospital, where the risk of financially motivated overtreatment is more acute.

False Claims

Misdemeanor penalties for false statements in pursuit of benefits were the first Medicare fraud laws. In the 1980s, criminal false claims enforcement was supplemented by an expanded and rewritten version of a Civil War procurement statute, the Civil False Claims Act.[17] This law imposed severe fines on violators and empowered private parties to bring qui tam cases in the name of the government and share in the financial recovery. Within a decade, Medicare claim submission forms were being used by both government antifraud enforcers and private whistle-blowers to allege multimillion-dollar offenses, sometimes including multiple violations of the False Claims Act during single episodes of care.

Although most false claims cases involved large institutions, such as hospitals and suppliers of medical equipment, even individual physicians face the threat of significant liability. In *United States* v. *Krizek*, the government spent six years pursuing an aging psychiatrist for upcoding office visits, and sought civil penalties of $81 million.[18] The defendant physician and his wife, who did his billing (while his lawyer daughter represented them), were refugees from both Nazi Germany and Soviet Russia, which reinforced the medical profession's perception of false claims enforcement as government persecution rather than deterrence of financial misconduct.[19]

In part because of its potential to reward private parties for uncovering fraud, false claims enforcement has been applied to a wider range of circumstances than other fraud and abuse laws have, producing greater uncertainty for the future as physicians and hospitals enter into new types of collaborations. In the 1990s, for example, both government and private enforcers urged courts to regard claims for payment involving medical services of inferior quality as false claims as a strategy for attacking restrictions imposed by managed care organizations and pharmacy benefit managers.[20]

The transition from paper to electronic claims processing complicates enforcement of the false claims laws because human agency is less easily traced and because batched processing renders ambiguous what constitutes a discrete claim to which a specified dollar fine would attach if false. Nonetheless, physicians are required to certify the accuracy of submitted claims in many instances, thereby explicitly assuming legal liability for falsity. This task may be much harder, and even arguably unfair, if the claim relates to a coordinated bundle of services provided by both professionals and institutions. Finally, as occurred during previous periods of rapid industry consolidation, integration, and changing affiliation, the coming wave of delivery system restructuring will expose new billing practices to a crowd of disgruntled employees and disenfranchised professionals who stand to gain emotionally and financially from *qui tam* litigation.

Incentives for Physicians to Withhold Necessary Services

The most significant change to the Medicare program between its original enactment and the addition of a prescription drug benefit in 2003 was the shift in 1983 from cost-plus reimbursement of hospitals to the Prospective Payment System (PPS) based on patient diagnosis (diagnosis-related groups, or DRGs). Lump-sum DRG payments, regardless of actual cost of care to the hospital, created an immediate rift between hospitals (which for the first time had an incentive to discharge patients at the earliest opportunity) and physicians (who benefited both financially and psychologically from patients remaining hospitalized until fully recovered). Because physician goodwill, and the referrals that flow from it, are a hospital's lifeblood, this financial tension provoked more bribery than bullying to alter physicians' mind-sets regarding inpatient length of stay. In response, Congress added a provision to existing fraud law that forbade hospitals from paying physicians to deny medically necessary services to patients.[21] This is commonly called the *civil monetary penalty* (CMP) law, although many other types of financial and clinical misconduct can give rise to civil fines.

Enforcement of the CMP law in the years following its enactment was occasional, and it attracted very little notice from lawyers or scholars. This changed in 1999, when the OIG was asked to evaluate the legality of physician-hospital gainsharing arrangements under the fraud and abuse laws. Commentators expected the enforcement agency to emphasize the risks of unlawful kickbacks and self-referral arising from revenue sharing within clinical departments. However, the OIG statement focused primarily on the civil monetary penalty law and construed hospital-based programs designed to alter clinical decisions in order to generate shared financial savings as unlawfully paying physicians to reduce or limit services.[22] Subsequent advisory opinions have approved both gainsharing and pay-for-performance (P4P) incentive arrangements under specific circumstances, but a general safe harbor for gainsharing does not yet exist.

Because clinical cost effectiveness will be the principal goal of future physician-hospital collaborations, participants are well advised to base their decisions on clear evidence that proposed practice changes will not reduce, and often will enhance, measurable quality of care. In addition, the OIG will need to modify its interpretation of the civil monetary penalty law to allow hospitals and physician groups latitude to reduce individual physician's discretion to use particularly expensive patient care items (for example, surgical implants). More generally, experience with the civil monetary penalty law should caution lawmakers about the danger of undercutting important new episode-based payment provisions that may accompany health reform by also enacting vague antifraud laws as safeguards.

Implications of Fraud and Abuse Law for Payment Reform

Because fraud and abuse law is an outgrowth of Medicare's fee-for-service payment policies, it will need to be changed dramatically if those payment policies are substantially altered to promote coordinated care delivery (see Chapters Three and Four). Historically, changes in fraud and abuse law have occurred periodically in response to new reimbursement methodologies. As noted, the civil monetary penalty statute was added to federal law as a direct result of Medicare's adopting prospective payment for hospitals, as were contemporaneous prohibitions on upcoding and unbundling. Managed care presented more systematic challenges, as contractual arrangements among providers and between providers and health plans created minimal risk of overcharging and overutilization (because overall

Medicare Advantage premiums were capped) but a somewhat greater risk of service denial or poor quality. Consequently, in 1993 the OIG proposed and Congress approved a new Stark exception for prepaid arrangements.

Episode-based payments of one type or another are likely to be developed as part of delivery system reform efforts in the coming years and probably can be accommodated by relatively straightforward parallel changes in fraud and abuse law. Transitional problems are certain to arise, however, if the same providers are paid for some services or some patients on a bundled basis and for others using traditional per service fees.

More interesting situations are likely to involve connections between the restructured primary care system and the specialty or acute care system, and between medical care as traditionally defined and population health. For example, will fraud and abuse law permit hospitals to pay office-based physicians for *medical home* services that prevent avoidable hospitalizations among their patients? What about so-called P4P4P—pay-for-performance for patients—payment made to *patients* to induce healthy behaviors and improve compliance with recommended preventive care? It remains to be seen whether these types of payment innovations will be welcomed by antifraud regulators as cost effective and health enhancing or resisted as exploitative or coercive of patients.

Tax Exemption

Laws limiting the structure and conduct of tax-exempt organizations constitute another legal challenge for physician-hospital collaboration. A majority of U.S. hospitals and a substantial number of HMOs and skilled nursing facilities are chartered as nonprofit corporations exempt from property and income taxes, including federal taxes if they meet standards contained in the Internal Revenue Code. In most instances, contributions to these entities are tax deductible, and many capital projects can be financed with low-interest, tax-exempt debt. The purpose of tax exemption is to encourage private investment in these activities, many of which further collective social purposes or serve individuals who cannot afford to pay. Surprisingly, the Internal Revenue Code lacks an explicit tax-exempt category for health care (unlike religion, science, and education), instead requiring such organizations to demonstrate that they meet general standards for charitable activities, as interpreted by the Internal Revenue Service (IRS) and the courts.

The law of tax-exempt organizations interacts with other laws affecting structural collaborations between physicians and hospitals. Most physician practices are organized for profit as sole proprietorships, regular or limited liability partnerships, or professional (including limited liability) corporations. Consequently, tax-exempt hospitals are not free to enter into many co-ownership arrangements with physicians, and may have their ability to employ physicians restricted by state corporate practice laws (described in the next section). However, if hospitals and physicians remain independent legal entities, transactions between them potentially face scrutiny for restraint of trade under Sherman Act § 1 (see the earlier discussion of antitrust law).

One would expect tax exemption and health care fraud laws to have synergistic policies, because both regimes are designed to prevent public funds from being diverted to benefit private parties. Indeed, public correspondence in the early 1990s between the chief counsels of the HHS OIG and the tax-exempt section of the IRS put hospitals on notice that fraudulent activity, such as payment of unlawful kickbacks, would also jeopardize their exempt status.[23] Nonetheless, conflicts between tax law and fraud law may arise in specific transactions. For example, tax law requires short contract terms in agreements between physicians and hospitals so that control over operations remains with the tax-exempt entity, whereas fraud law favors longer terms because brief ones allow the parties to adjust compensation at each renewal date to reward referrals or other favoritism during the prior term.

Two issues dominate legal scrutiny of tax-exempt organizations: community benefit and private inurement. Each issue is explained in the next section, and special considerations related to physician-hospital collaboration are discussed.

Community Benefit Standards

Federally tax-exempt organizations must be "organized and operated exclusively" for specific activities of benefit to the community.[24] One aspect of tax exemption enforcement involves defining the activities that qualify as community benefit and whether (and how) to enforce a minimum quantitative standard. Traditional metrics under federal law were maintenance of an emergency department, an open medical staff (itself perhaps a historical source of operating inefficiency), and willingness to treat uninsured and publicly insured (Medicare and Medicaid) patients. To accommodate changes in these hospital practices in the 1970s, the IRS began to treat community benefit standards flexibly, but concern over abuses mounted as cost pressures on hospitals intensified in subsequent decades. Recently, these soft metrics have been supplemented by state and federal laws requiring more detailed public reporting of nonprofit operations, including quantitative measures of free or discounted care.[25] Such rules do not specify a minimum amount needed to justify a hospital's charitable exemptions, but cases presenting this issue continue to be litigated in state courts over property and state income tax liability.

Private Inurement, Private Benefit, and Excess Benefit Transactions

At the heart of federal tax policy is the prohibition on any part of the net earnings of a tax-exempt organization accruing to private controlling parties, whether or not they are formally owners. Unlawful profit sharing is termed private inurement, and constitutes a serious offense, even in small amounts.[26] To police inurement more effectively, the IRS now has the authority to impose large excise taxes on controlling persons who receive unlawful profits, also called excess benefits.[27] This creates a more credible deterrent than the draconian remedy of cancelling a hospital's tax exemption and rendering its outstanding bond indebtedness retroactively taxable to the holders.

To make matters even more complicated, private inurement is a different concept from private benefit, which is an inevitable aspect of operating a hospital in which private physicians care for patients using the hospital's tax-exempt facilities. Private benefit is permitted in small amounts, but hospitals cannot offer physicians free office space or other substantial perks (which would also be prohibited by fraud and abuse law).

In addition, the "organized and operated" condition for federal tax exemption implies that control over operations must be retained by a nonprofit hospital's governing body and not be ceded contractually to a profit-making management corporation regardless of the hospital's need to improve efficiency.[28] As described in the next section, joint ventures that utilize tax-exempt assets are similarly constrained. Decisions to create parent (holding) companies to coordinate the activities of several tax-exempt hospitals may also be restricted, although federal law has been modified over the years to allow nonprofit parents that are not operating companies to qualify as public charities for tax purposes. (State law may still limit mergers and affiliations involving nonprofit hospitals if services would no longer be available in the localities specified by the participating institutions' charter documents.)

Implications of Tax Exemption Law for Payment Reform and Coverage Expansion

Gainsharing and other clinical joint ventures between physicians and tax-exempt hospitals must be carefully structured to avoid legal challenge. Physicians on a hospital's medical staff were for many years automatically deemed insiders (and therefore *controlling parties*) because of their profound influence over hospital policy, potentially subjecting the hospital to private inurement violations in any transaction involving them. However, the IRS position on physicians as insiders was changed in the 1990s in recognition of the increased sophistication of hospital management. Still, these tax considerations imply that caution must be exercised to avoid explicit profit sharing between hospitals and physicians in gainsharing programs, as well as the assignment to physicians of governance roles in hospital operations. Moreover, the private benefit conferred on physicians by participating in the hospital's clinical operations must be no more than incidental to the public benefit achieved.

Bundled payment methodologies designed to improve physician-hospital collaboration would be most easily administered through direct physician employment by hospitals or indirect employment by creation of a newly defined, nonprofit form of ACO. As a practical matter, however, this degree of structural uniformity in the health care system seems implausible in the next few years. Because bundled payments would not allay the tax law's concern over diverting charitable subsidies away from the exempt entity, acceptable forms of revenue sharing by hospitals with nonemployed physicians may need to be specified in amendments to federal tax law.

If health insurance coverage is significantly expanded by federal law, it will become important to move beyond individual charity as the touchstone for compliance with nonprofit hospitals' tax obligations (or, for that matter, physicians' professional ethical obligations). Epidemic chronic disease from unhealthy lifestyles highlights the importance of incorporating prevention and public health into medical care to a much greater extent than previously. Redefining community benefit to emphasize investment in these public goods by hospitals and physicians working together would be a productive direction for tax law. For example, tax-exempt entities offering high-quality, low-unit-cost orthopedic services could fulfill their charitable obligations by promoting weight reduction in their communities as well as by providing surgical services to the residual population of uninsured individuals.

State Laws

For about a century, the U.S. medical profession has steered a delicate course between the Scylla of control by government and the Charybdis of control by corporations. Political battles over government control are fought primarily at the federal level because so many federal dollars flow through Medicare to health care providers. Political battles over corporate control (as well as turf wars among organized professions) are fought mainly at the state level because state police powers have traditionally governed licensing of health professionals and health care institutions.

These historical patterns, plus various constitutional constraints, suggest that a frontal assault using federal law to eliminate state law barriers to provider collaboration would be ill advised in most cases. Direct strategies to change the federalist balance succeed only in rare paradigm shifts when the underlying theory of government regulation as it is understood by the public changes dramatically, and only when the new theory also coincides with perceived financial and scientific advantages at the federal level. Automobile safety, for example, largely shifted from state to federal oversight in the 1960s because vehicle and highway design supplanted lack of driver discipline as the scientific explanation for crashes, and because the visible success of the space program (and the Eisenhower interstate highway system) reinforced public confidence in federal engineering.[29] Absent a sense of national solidarity regarding health insurance, medical care, and wellness, there seems to be little evidence of an equivalent phenomenon in health care.[30] To the contrary, health care tends to provoke a localist bias similar to that found for education.

A number of state laws affect hospitals' and physicians' ability to improve collaboration. Only a sampling of such laws are included here: health professional licensing and scope of practice, the corporate practice of medicine doctrine and physician employment, medical staff credentialing, insurance regulation, and medical malpractice. Each of these areas of law is described in the following sections, and special considerations related to physician-hospital collaboration are discussed.

Health Professional Licensing and Scope of Practice

Improving health care delivery requires deploying health professionals with different skills in different combinations than has been conventional. One objective is to have basic services performed by the most affordable, and therefore most accessible, individuals who are qualified to do so. A second objective is to improve coordination of care for patients who require sophisticated treatments for serious or multiple diseases. Professional licensing has a long and established history as an exercise of state government's general police powers to protect health and safety and was validated as constitutional by the U.S. Supreme Court in the late nineteenth century.[31] For nearly as long, licensing also has been criticized as an economically motivated practice that confers exclusive practice privileges on politically organized groups of providers, allows them broad self-regulatory discretion to keep their numbers small and prices high, discourages innovative collaborations, and prevents consumers from accessing less elite but cheaper services.

State licensing programs have proliferated in response to the development of new medical technologies, the increased availability of health insurance to fund services, and the resurgence of public interest in complementary and alternative healing. Most states currently license dozens of health professions, ranging from perfusionists to naturopaths. Physicians occupy a unique position atop this hierarchy. They possess an expansive right to practice medicine, while others who do so without explicit statutory protection commit a serious crime. Nonphysician health professionals have their authorized tasks specifically and narrowly defined, often with an additional requirement of physician supervision.[32]

The debate over patient-centered medical homes and retail medical clinics as sources of improved primary care encapsulates the licensing issues involved in practice reorganization. The medical profession tends to criticize retail clinics, which are usually staffed by nurse practitioners, as perpetuating fragmented care, and it argues that, instead, physicians should be paid for providing comprehensive medical home services. But physicians demand higher prices for their time than many can afford to pay for basic services, whereas care coordination can be achieved through institutional processes as well as through independent physician direction. Moreover, improving access can often be accomplished more rapidly by expanding the nonphysician workforce, which undergoes far shorter and less expensive training periods than do physicians.

Under current law, however, inexpensive nonphysician care is viable only in states that include such services within the authorized scope of practice of the relevant individuals (advanced practice nurses, physician assistants, and so on) and that do not impose large additional cost burdens by requiring physician supervision to be on-site or limited to very few supervisees. Yet attempts to change these laws provoke fierce physician resistance. This legal uncertainty and contentiousness further increases costs and curtails innovation by discouraging schools from expanding nonphysician training programs. In addition, physicians may be reluctant to support novel practice arrangements even if they remain in charge for fear of provoking a punitive response from the disciplinary arms of state medical boards.

Because Medicare reimbursement defers to state licensing laws, major provider payment reforms that could encourage physician-hospital collaboration may be hampered if state scope of practice laws limit the ability to offer cost-effective services or if the necessary aggregate workforce is unavailable. Financial incentives to alter practice laws in order to receive federal funds may help to relieve the former concern, and expanded federal support for nonphysician primary care training programs may help to address the latter.

A more extreme approach would be to include within episode-based payment reforms a program of institutional licensure, under which each Medicare-certified institutional provider would have significant leeway to assemble care using both professional and nonprofessional skills, and would report and publicly disclose the processes it uses and the outcomes it achieves. More broadly, measuring the quality of services in similar fashion for different primary care professionals will be very important.

The Corporate Practice of Medicine and Physician Employment

State restrictions on the corporate practice of medicine bear special mention because of their potential effects on both physician-hospital collaborations and the organization of so-called focused factories for the standardized delivery of efficient, high-quality inpatient and specialty care. The legal underpinning of corporate practice restrictions is straightforward (if contestable on normative grounds): corporations cannot practice medicine because only individuals can meet the educational, testing, and character-related prerequisites for licensure. However, the practical import of the corporate practice doctrine has been to prohibit or limit the employment of physicians by corporate entities, sometimes including hospitals. The legal source (statute or judicial decision) and scope of the doctrine (all corporations or only for-profit corporations not licensed as institutional providers) vary widely from state to state.

Fewer than ten states actively enforce such laws, but California, Illinois, New York, Ohio, and Texas are among them.[33] In these states, corporate practice limitations directly affect potential episode-based payment programs and transparency initiatives because they restrict the ways in which physicians and hospitals can organize themselves for both payment and accountability. Workarounds exist, notably foundation models for structuring large multispecialty practices (see Chapter Seven) and long-term contractual relationships between hospitals and their affiliated physicians. However, these structures add cost, decrease flexibility, and create uncertainty for the contracting parties.

Even where employment is permissible, employed physicians may receive special legal solicitude. State patient protection legislation in the 1990s, for example, sometimes included statutory protections for physicians acting as whistle-blowers against overreaching by managed care organizations or otherwise "advocating" for good patient care.[34] These laws are not problematic on their face but can be used by disenchanted individuals to deter or delay productive changes in methods of health care delivery.

Medical Staff Credentialing

The legal basis for the open, voluntary credentialing and affiliation process by which hospitals typically populate their facilities with physicians has profound implications for the cost, quality, and efficiency of medical care. Credentialing is the process by which a hospital, acting through its existing medical staff of affiliated but otherwise independent physicians, verifies the qualifications of new applicants and grants them privileges to admit patients and to perform specific procedures. U.S. physicians enjoy an unusual degree of freedom to treat patients in advanced hospital settings while also maintaining both their formal independence and their private offices or clinics.

The relationship between hospitals and their medical staffs is governed primarily by state law, although specific credentialing procedures are based on accreditation requirements from the Joint Commission.[35] Peer review privileges and immunities (including from federal antitrust liability) are conferred by both state law and the federal Health Care Quality Improvement Act of 1986, which also improved information exchange among licensing and credentialing bodies by creating the National Practitioner Data Bank.[36] These laws continue to partition general hospital administration from oversight of clinical quality, with the latter function assigned to the physicians, most of them in private practice, who use hospital facilities.

Self-governing medical staffs are deeply ingrained in professional culture and state law. Most medical staff governance plays a constructive role in assuring quality and promoting cooperation among physicians. Moreover, credentialing laws (sometimes in combination with antitrust law) have accommodated many important changes in physician-hospital affiliation practices, such as denying staff privileges to unqualified applicants, consolidating hospital departments through exclusive contracts (for example, emergency medicine, radiology, anesthesiology), and shifting large amounts of inpatient care to dedicated hospitalists.

However, certain aspects of staff relations remain controversial and may influence efforts to reinvent hospital-based care delivery. One issue that relates to transparency initiatives is how quality should be assessed in credentialing decisions, particular when adverse actions are based on statistical measurement and benchmarking, as opposed to evidence of specific clinical errors. Another issue is the use of *economic credentialing*, in which medical staff decisions are based on the revenue generated by physicians as well as the quality achieved. A third issue, *conflicts credentialing*, has arisen mainly in connection with physician-owned specialty hospitals and involves the degree to which general hospitals can require affiliated physicians to be loyal business partners (not diverting patients elsewhere) as well as competent ones. Each of these situations has provoked varying legal responses at the state and federal levels.

Insurance Regulation

Insurance, including health insurance, is nearly always governed by state rather than federal law. Furthermore, several states have created dedicated administrative agencies to oversee HMOs and other forms of managed care. In California, for example, Knox-Keene plans (the state's term for HMOs) were under the purview of the state Department of Corporations, not the Department of Insurance, until a separate Department of Managed Health Care was formed. Whether or not HMOs are regulated separately from insurers, laws enacted by many states during the managed care backlash of the late 1990s continue to subject contracting practices between payers and providers to a host of requirements and restrictions. Most of these laws are applicable even to coverage sponsored by self-insured employers, notwithstanding the important preemptive effects of the federal Employee Retirement Income Security Act (ERISA).[37]

Managed care is seldom mentioned by the current generation of health care reformers, undoubtedly because of its unpopularity with both physicians and the public. However, the failings of the U.S. health care system are largely attributable to persistently unmanaged care, and the vast majority of reforms designed to improve clinical cost effectiveness either duplicate or refine the strategies that dominated managed care a decade ago. These include placing providers at financial risk for the cost of services, channeling expensive treatments to preferred providers, improving prevention and management of chronic disease, and giving patients incentives to seek only necessary care. Although the evidence base and actuarial science underlying these maneuvers has improved since the 1990s, with more explicit attention to quality effects, they present similar risks of claims denials and undertreatment. Moreover, many network-model HMOs have collapsed because of legal restrictions and continuing cost pressures, leaving less integrated insurance products such as preferred provider organizations (PPOs) as the basis for future reforms.

Existing managed care and insurance laws may interact unpredictably with initiatives to improve health care delivery through physician-hospital collaboration. For example, some forms of episode-based payment may place providers at sufficient financial risk as to be regulated by states for solvency as insurers. Similarly, state PPO regulations may deter efforts to create tiered coverage of physicians and hospitals based on rankings of quality or cost effectiveness.

Medical Malpractice

Another very important area of state law is medical malpractice, which carries tremendous economic and symbolic importance for physicians. Although tort reformers periodically attempt to alter medical malpractice liability through federal legislation, the localized nature of patient injury, the established patterns of negotiation between plaintiffs' lawyers and state-based malpractice insurers, and the impracticality of shifting such widespread litigation to the federal docket all serve to keep malpractice as primarily a state issue. Malpractice is far too complicated a subject to address comprehensively in this chapter. However, a few observations regarding its influence on hospital-physician collaboration are important.

Malpractice risks are central to physician-hospital integration and collaboration. Hospitals are potential deep pockets in most serious malpractice cases, and state standards for holding them liable on theories of actual agency, apparent agency, or corporate negligence vary widely. Changing payment arrangements and practice structures can easily alter the associated liability risks, especially because decisions in litigation are typically made by local trial courts that enjoy substantial discretion.

Physicians and hospitals are also subject to various state (and some National Practitioner Data Bank) requirements regarding reporting and potential public disclosure of malpractice suits and settlements. Depending on the specifics of reporting and the extent and form of collaboration between physicians and hospitals, complying with these requirements can be controversial because of the risks to professional reputations. Unfamiliar methods of provider payment can also increase liability risks, as occurred in the 1990s when capitation and other financial incentives under managed care were framed by litigants as violations of physicians' fiduciary duty of loyalty to patients. At a more practical level, hospitals and physicians may wish to share malpractice insurance costs in ways not obviously permissible under fraud and abuse law, or to bind patients to less adversarial forms of dispute resolution (for example, arbitration or mediation).

Implications of State Laws for Health Reform

Unless public sentiment turns overwhelmingly toward sweeping federalization of the health care system, state law issues will be central to delivery system restructuring even if significant health reform legislation is enacted by Congress. At the moment, it seems unlikely that the Obama administration's health reform efforts can generate a paradigm shift connected to practice organization, information, wellness, patient safety, or cost control. Faith in large government projects is not particularly high even if new theories of success—including those explored in this book—come to be widely accepted.

Consequently, federal influence may be most effectively expanded through conditional subsidy and indirect oversight. Medicare payment policies that assure funding for basic care not provided by physicians or that bundle payment for specialized care by institutional and individual providers create strong incentives for facilitative changes in state law. Similarly, expanded federal programs for public reporting of provider quality and price or for electronic information exchange among providers may encourage change in regressive aspects of professionally controlled state laws. These strategies are particularly important for two hot-button issues around which physicians have long been engaged in interprofessional political warfare at the state level: malpractice liability (against trial lawyers) and scope of professional practice (involving rival health professions).

Regarding malpractice law, federal health care reform offers an opportunity to reconcile state law with a new paradigm for patient safety and quality improvement based on practice integration, evidence-based medicine, and institutional accountability. However, one cannot overstate the importance of getting the symbolism right when it comes to malpractice policy. Physicians engage with malpractice liability primarily as an issue of control. Physicians resent malpractice suits because they seem to be random attacks, motivated mainly by financial opportunism, that trap unlucky doctors in a Kafkaesque nightmare of emotional stress, career disruption, and arbitrary decision making. As a result, physicians display strong preferences for familiar malpractice reforms, notably caps on non-economic damages and limits on attorney fees. Even if physicians overcome their suspicion that more sweeping changes to the malpractice system are merely a trick of the trial lawyers, they may still be fearful that the cure will leave them even less control over their professional lives than the disease.

For this reason, the Clinton Administration's tentative proposal that malpractice liability be shifted from physicians to health plans was seen by the medical profession as horrifying confirmation that managed care organizations would dictate clinical practices in a reformed health care system, rather than as a conceptually logical measure to moderate health plans' incentives to cut costs by holding them accountable for quality as well. The Obama Administration faces analogous risks that intellectually attractive malpractice reform proposals will provoke unpleasant visceral reactions from physicians. For example, reformers might reasonably wish to make the federal government financially responsible for malpractice suits by deeming physicians participating in new public programs (such as the much-debated public option) to be federal employees covered by the Federal Tort Claims Act. However, this change might be perceived by the medical profession as evidence of a presidential plan for socialized medicine. Alternatively, an effort to immunize physicians from suits based on compliance with government guidelines for medical practice might be seen as a step down the road to rationing.

Conclusion

Law is a pervasive feature of the U.S. health care system, and any major effort to redesign the delivery of medical services must evaluate the legal environment for both barriers and opportunities. As this chapter has illustrated, current health law is far from seamless in its application to potential improvements in the organization and performance of the health care delivery system. Tensions already exist among various sources of law, which sends mixed signals to health care reformers. Moreover, law is not only complex but also uncertain, which adds to the business and personal risk of restructuring current practices. Particularly for physicians, the perceived risk depends in large part on whether legal enforcement is channeled through professional regulatory processes, general government oversight, or private lawsuits.

As health reform proceeds, the following key questions regarding the legal environment should guide the debate:

1. What legal changes would remove current disincentives for the desired delivery system transformation?
2. What legal changes would provide new positive incentives for that transformation?
3. What legal changes are needed to reduce defensive behavior by health care providers and other stakeholders during a transitional period from the current delivery system to a transformed one?
4. What legal changes are needed to prevent the leakage of undesirable behavior from regulated sectors to sectors that are temporarily or permanently unregulated (for example, insurers or providers selecting low-risk patients for programs in which their performance will be measured and shunting high-risk patients to unmeasured activities)?
5. What legal changes are needed to prevent the spillover of behaviors that are beneficial when conducted in regulated sectors into unregulated sectors where they may be harmful (for example, physician-hospital collaborations that facilitate price-fixing)?

Because federal health reform legislation has emphasized expansions of insurance coverage rather than restructuring of the health care delivery system, federal health regulatory agencies should evaluate their existing enforcement approaches for potential barriers to physician-hospital collaboration, modify discretionary policies that appear problematic, and seek congressional approval of changes requiring statutory authorization. Specifically, systematic evaluation of antikickback, self-referral, civil monetary penalty, and tax exemption standards should be performed at the earliest opportunity, as the administrative agencies responsible for enforcing these laws are accustomed to altering their policies collaboratively in response to new payment methods and provider structures.

There does not appear to be a pressing need to revisit federal antitrust law, but any comprehensive federal endorsement of new health care delivery models such as patient-centered medical homes and ACOs should pay explicit attention to the anticompetitive risks associated with those models. Antitrust enforcers and counselors should also provide sufficient guidance to the health care community so that providers will understand how they can undertake innovative approaches to health care delivery—including collaborative approaches by hospitals and physicians—without undue antitrust risk.

Notes

1. Additional details about antitrust and fraud and abuse risks are presented in R. F. Leibenluft, J. L. Diesenhaus, E. M. Bain, and L. L. Oliver, "Hospital-Physician Collaborations: Antitrust and Health Care Fraud and Abuse Considerations," in *2009 Health Law Handbook*, ed. A. G. Gosfield, 251–99 (St. Paul, MN: Thomson West, 2009).

2. For reasons of space, this chapter omits many federal and state laws relevant to health care reform, including the Emergency Medical Treatment and Active Labor Act of 1986 (EMTALA), the Employment Retirement Income Security Act of 1974 (ERISA), the Americans with Disabilities Act (ADA), the Health Insurance Portability and Accountability Act of 1996 (HIPAA), federal research regulations, facilities licensing, consumer protection, and public health.

3. *FTC* v. *Indiana Federation of Dentists*, 476 U.S. 447 (1986); *Jefferson Parish Hospital District* v. *Hyde*, 466 U.S. 2 (1984); *Arizona* v. *Maricopa County Medical Society*, 457 U.S. 332 (1982); *National Society of Professional Engineers* v. *United States*, 435 U.S. 679 (1978); *Goldfarb* v. *Virginia State Bar*, 421 U.S. 773 (1975).

4. P. J. Hammer and W. M. Sage, "Antitrust, Health Care Quality, and the Courts," *Columbia Law Review* 102, no. 3 (2002): 545–649.

5. Following several earlier victories, government antitrust enforcers brought and lost seven challenges to hospital mergers: *California* v. *Sutter Health System*, 84 F. Supp. 2d 1057 (N.D. Cal. 2000) (Oakland, CA); *Tenet Healthcare Corporation* v. *FTC*, 186 F.3d 1045 (8th Cir. 1999) (Poplar Bluff, MO); *United States* v. *Long Island Jewish Medical Center*, 983 F. Supp. 121 (E.D.N.Y. 1997) (Nassau County, NY); *FTC* v. *Butterworth Health Corp.*, 946 F. Supp. 1285 (W.D. Mich 1996) (Grand Rapids, MI); *United States* v. *Mercy Health Services*, 902 F. Supp. 968 (N.D. Iowa 1995) (Dubuque, IA); *FTC* v. *Freeman Hospital*, 911 F.Supp;. 1213 (W.D. Mo.), aff'd, 69 F.3 260 (8th Cir. 1995) (Joplin, MO); *FTC* v. *Hospital Board of Directors of Lee County*, 1994-1 Trade Cas. ¶ 70,593 (M.D. Fla.); aff'd, 38 F.3d 1184 (11th Cir. 1994) (Lee County, FL). In 2007, a Federal Trade Commission ruling finally resulted in another government win: in the Matter of Evanston Northwestern Healthcare Group and ENH Medical Group, Inc., File No. 011 0234 (issued August 6, 2007), http://www.ftc.gov/os/adjpro/d9315/070806opinion.pdf (Highland Park, IL).

6. *Professional Real Estate Investors, Inc.* v. *Columbia Pictures Industries, Inc.*, 508 U.S. 49 (1993).

7. 15 *U.S. Code* § 1.

8. U.S. Department of Justice and Federal Trade Commission (FTC), *Antitrust Guidelines for Collaborations Among Competitors* (2000), at 8, http://www.ftc.gov/os/2000/04/ftcdojguidelines.pdf. This chapter refers to these guidelines and to the DOJ and FTC's industry-specific *Statements of Antitrust Enforcement Policy in Health Care* (1996), http://www.usdoj.gov/atr/public/guidelines/0000.pdf,

because they reflect how the federal antitrust agencies interpret and intend to apply the antitrust laws. Although not binding on the courts, conduct that is consistent with these guidelines will likely be difficult to challenge successfully.

9. Compare FTC Advisory Opinion re MedSouth, Inc., http://www.ftc.gov/bc/adops/medsouth.shtm; FTC Advisory Opinion re Greater Rochester Independent Practice Association, http://www.ftc.gov/bc/adops/gripa.pdf; and FTC Advisory Opinion re TriState Health Partners, Inc., http://www.ftc.gov/os/closings/staff/090413tristateaoletter.pdf (favorable advisory opinions) with FTC Advisory Opinion re Suburban Health Organization, http://www.ftc.gov/opa/2006/03/shor31.shtm (unfavorable advisory opinion).

10. T. B. Leary, R. F. Leibenluft, S. A. Pozen, and T. E. Weir, *Guidance on Clinical Integration* (working paper, Hogan and Hartson LLP for the American Hospital Association, 2007), http://www.aha.org/aha/content/2007/pdf/070417clinicalintegration.pdf.

11. For a discussion of ancillarity in the context of clinical integration, see R. F. Leibenluft and T. E. Weir, "Clinical Integration: Assessing the Antitrust Issues," in *Health Law Handbook*, ed. A. G. Gosfield, 32–24 (St. Paul, MN: Thomson West, 2004).

12. In the FTC advisory opinions, one rationale for joint negotiations that has been accepted is the need to have a consistent panel of providers participating in the collaboration's initiatives, providers who can cross-refer to each other with respect to all patients and regardless of payer. This can be assured only through joint negotiations, so that when the collaboration signs up with a particular health plan, it does so on behalf of all member providers.

13. Oct. 30, 1972, Public Law 92-603, Title II, §§ 242(c), 278(b)(9), 86 *U.S. Statutes at Large* 1419, 1454.

14. 42 *U.S. Code* § 1320a-7b(b).

15. Medicare demonstration projects to permit gainsharing arrangements: Act of Feb. 8, 2006 (Deficit Reduction Act of 2005), Public Law 109-171, Title V, Subtitle A, § 5007.

16. Dec. 19, 1989, Public Law 101-239, Title VI, Subtitle A, Part 3, Subpart A, § 6204(a), 103 *U.S. Statutes at Large* 2236; Aug. 10, 1993 (Omnibus Budget Reconciliation Act of 1993), Public Law 103-66, Title XIII, Ch 2, Subch A, Part III, § 13562(a), 107 *U.S. Statutes at Large* 596. The current law is codified at 42 *U.S. Code* § 1395nn.

17. 31 *U.S. Code* § 3729–3731.

18. *United States* v. *Krizek*, 192 F.3d 1024 (D.C. Cir. 1999).

19. See T. L. Greaney and J. H. Krause, "*United States* v. *Krizek:* Rough Justice Under the Civil False Claims Act," in *Health Law and Bioethics: Cases in Context*, ed. S. Johnson, J. Krause, R. Saver, and R. Wilson (New York: Aspen, 2009).

20. For example, *United States ex rel. Mikes* v. *Straus*, 274 F.3d 687 (2d Cir. 2001) (rejecting a false claim suit involving quality of spirometry testing).

21. 42 *U.S. Code* § 1320a-7a(b).

22. "Gainsharing Arrangements and CMPs for Hospital Payments to Physicians to Reduce or Limit Services to Beneficiaries," 64 *Federal Register* 37, 985 (July 14, 1999).

23. "HHS' Thornton Writes IRS' Sullivan," *Exempt Organization Tax Review* 7 (1993), 705.

24. 26 *U.S. Code* § 501(c)(3).

25. In 2007, for example, the IRS mandated a Community Benefit Report (Schedule H) from nonprofit hospitals in conjunction with their annual Form 990 filing.

26. See IRS General Counsel Memorandum 39862 (Dec. 2, 1991) (analyzing net revenue stream joint ventures between physicians and hospitals).

27. 26 *U.S. Code* § 4958.

28. See, for example, *St. David's Health Care System* v. *United States*, 349 F.3d 232 (5th Cir. 2003).

29. J. L. Mashaw and D. L. Harfst, *The Struggle for Auto Safety* (Cambridge, MA: Harvard University Press, 1990).

30. See W. M. Sage, "Solidarity: Unfashionable, But Still American," in *Connecting American Values to National Health Care Reform*, ed. T. H. Murray, 10–12 (Garrison, NY: Hastings Center, 2009).

31. *Dent* v. *West Virginia*, 129 U.S. 114 (1889).

32. In Texas, each day of practicing medicine without a valid license is a third-degree felony: *Texas Occupations Code* (Medical Practice Act) § 165.152.

33. For example, *Texas Occupations Code* § 164.052.

34. *California Business and Professions Code* § 2056(a).

35. The Joint Commission was formerly known as the Joint Commission on Accreditation of Healthcare Organizations.

36. Act of Nov. 14, 1986, Public Law 99-660, codified at 42 *U.S. Code* § 11101.

37. See *Rush Prudential HMO, Inc.* v. *Moran*, 536 U.S. 355 (2002).

CHAPTER SEVEN

OVERCOMING BARRIERS TO IMPROVED COLLABORATION AND ALIGNMENT

Governance Issues

Jeffrey A. Alexander
Gary J. Young
Commentaries by James A. DeNuccio and John R. Combes

Introduction

This chapter is concerned with the role of hospital and medical staff governance in strengthening the alignment of hospitals and physicians for the purpose of improving the quality, efficiency, and accessibility of health care services. The governance of these entities is critical to the improvement of health care services in the United States because it is where the policymaking and oversight responsibilities for hospitals lie. This chapter focuses on governance of non-profit, community hospitals, which make up the majority of general hospitals in the United States.[1] Hospital boards have not traditionally played a significant role in managing hospitals' relationships with their medical staffs. However, some have argued that increased levels of competition and discord between hospital management and physicians provide an opportunity for boards and medical staff leadership to establish new structures, cultures of collaboration and cooperation, and common incentives to improve quality and reduce costs.[2] Hospital boards represent their communities, and to the extent that the community desires improvement in patient experiences across the continuum of care, the board can and should play a role in shaping hospital attitudes and behaviors toward the medical staff (and vice versa) to achieve these ends.[3] Similarly, medical staffs may have the opportunity in the future to collectively shape the policies and operations of institutions to the mutual benefit of hospitals and physicians. These idealized goals notwithstanding, a number of governance challenges—cultural, structural, historical, and regulatory—will have to be addressed before this can happen.

The process of hospital governance is distinguished from that of management or supervision. It involves setting goals and developing strategy for their achievement, using the structure of a board of trustees or directors to which top administrative officers and the chief of the medical staff of the organization report.[4] This description of hospital governance reflects current, prescribed roles of boards, but does not account for the development of governance structures over time or the unique challenges faced by boards in carrying out these responsibilities. Indeed, the role of governing bodies in American hospitals has evolved over the course of history in response to environmental, structural, and technological changes.[5]

This chapter reviews the historical development of hospital governing boards and medical staffs and how regulation, reimbursement, and competition have shaped relations between the two groups. It then considers issues and problems with hospital governing boards and hospital medical staffs and possible future directions in hospital and medical staff governance to promote alignment. Finally, it provides a set of recommended strategies to enable hospital and medical staff governing entities to take a leading role in promoting alignment between hospitals and physicians.

Historical Development of Modern Hospital Governance

The original hospitals were charitable, nonprofit institutions that existed to care for the poor.[6] These early hospitals relied on donations to operate. Accordingly, governing boards were composed of elite members of the community who were effective in soliciting funds for the hospital and who also served as managers. One of their responsibilities, for example, was to assess neediness of potential patients and make admissions decisions accordingly. In the early part of the twentieth century the financial success of hospitals became dependent on physicians who practiced there, which gave the medical staff power within the organization they did not previously hold.[7] The board's power diminished as its contribution to the financial position of the hospital became less significant. Trustees during this period began to serve only legitimizing roles, symbolically tying the community to the hospital when they had previously served as ultimate leaders of the institution.

The history of the governing board in modern hospitals can effectively be divided into three periods, described in the following sections.

Peaceful Coexistence: Dual Lines of Authority in the Hospital

The first historical period comprises the majority of the twentieth century, during which private nonprofit hospitals in the United States acted as independent entities governed by boards of influential local residents. Although hospitals competed for the allegiance of physicians, primarily by promoting quality and technological sophistication of services and equipment available in the hospital, there was little direct competition for patients. For most of this period, hospitals and physicians did not advertise their services to patients, thus reducing the potential for competition.

Generally, hospitals did not employ practicing physicians. In fact, during the first half of the twentieth century, twenty-six states passed corporate practice of medicine laws that prohibited hospitals and other corporate entities governed by nonphysicians from employing physicians (see Chapter Six). Instead, physicians cared for their patients in hospitals as attending physicians, after being granted hospital admitting privileges. As described in Chapter Two, during this time, the hospital was seen as the physicians' workshop. A combination of regulations and mutual interest based on common economic incentives allowed hospital governing boards and physician medical staffs to remain separate and only loosely connected.[8] Also important, coordination and oversight of a physician's work in the hospital was performed by the medical staff themselves, in a process known as self-governance, while other activities performed by employed hospital personnel were coordinated and managed within the hospital's administrative structure. These dual lines of authority provided the hospital and its attending physicians with a structure through which their work could be coordinated, while buffering physicians from bureaucratic control. Essentially, this parallel governance structure was functional under the payment systems of this era—fee-for-service (FFS)—because both hospitals and medical staff members gained by admitting more patients and performing more procedures. Under such financial incentives, integrated governance and tight coordination were unnecessary.

Although the dual administrative–medical staff governance structure has long been a key characteristic of modern hospitals in the United States, separation of authority and responsibility along these two lines of professional activity has not fully insulated each party from the actions of the other. For example, even though medical staff are typically independent contractors to the hospital, the hospital board itself can be held legally responsible for errors that medical staff members make. This was reinforced in the case of *Darling* v. *Charleston Community Hospital* in the 1960s, when the Illinois Supreme Court ruled that the hospital board was ultimately responsible for ensuring competency of physicians to whom it extended medical staff appointment and clinical privileges. Thus, though dual lines of authority worked well under FFS, the Darling case began to expose cracks in the system and set the stage for the erosion of hospital-physician alignment in the late twentieth and early twenty-first centuries.

Troubled Waters: Changes In Reimbursement, Regulation, and Competition

The second historical period, beginning in the early 1980s, was marked by several developments that placed hospitals and physicians in an increasingly strained and uncertain relationship, thereby significantly weakening the dual lines of authority structure.[9] One development was the adoption by public and private payers of prospective payment systems for health care providers that were intended to contain escalating costs (see Chapters Two and Four). These systems impose fixed prices or budgets on providers so that they have a financial incentive to control patient care costs. However, these systems also can throw hospital and physician incentives out of alignment. At the time the federal government shifted from a cost-based to a Prospective Payment System for hospitals participating in the Medicare program, Medicare and most other payers continued to reimburse physicians on a fee-for-service basis that, in principle, encouraged physicians to provide more services during the course of a patient admission, even while hospitals had an incentive to provide less.

Another development was the emergence of strong competitive pressures on health care providers for patients. For example, managed care plans began to contract selectively with hospitals and physicians, creating competition among providers for insurance contracts.[10] Many states moved toward deregulating health care through the elimination of controls on hospital construction and prices, which further fostered competitive pressures to acquire the latest technology, build the most elaborate facilities, and engage in strategies to acquire market share from other hospitals in the area.[11] In the absence of regulatory controls, hospitals became more aggressive in offering new services, particularly those with high profit margins. Also, for the first time, hospitals formed marketing departments to promote themselves. However, this competitive orientation among providers forced hospitals and their medical staff to reconsider the nature of their relationship and whether and under what circumstances closer collaboration would be mutually beneficial.

A third key development during this time was the availability of new technologies that enabled physicians to provide many formerly hospital-based services on an outpatient basis. For some types of physician specialists, this development reduced their dependence on the hospital, as they could now perform certain procedures in their own offices or free-standing ambulatory clinics.

In the presence of these developments relating to reimbursement, regulation, and competition, hospital governing boards began to assume a much stronger business orientation in both appearance and behavior, which had direct implications for the hospital–medical staff relationship.[12] During the 1980s, the trend among hospital boards appeared to be toward fewer members and stronger insider representation from the medical staff.[13] In theory, smaller boards facilitated faster decision making, whereas stronger representation from the medical staff served two major objectives: (1) it promoted better board decision making through the input of physicians who carry valuable knowledge about hospital operations from their vantage point on the front lines of patient care; and (2) it allowed for the co-optation of physicians, important hospital stakeholders, by incorporating them into the governance structure.[14] Additionally, hospital boards created new forms of organization to align the interests of the hospital and its physicians. These organizational arrangements, which include physician hospital organizations (PHOs), management service organizations (MSOs), foundation models, and integrated delivery systems (IDSs), tend to be formally structured, contractual, or corporate in character and to include physicians outside the formal membership of the medical staff.[15] For example, physician hospital organizations are organized to facilitate joint contracting with managed care organizations and generally entail professional services agreements with physician groups and separate incorporation from the hospital and physician group. Beyond their structural features, these organizational arrangements require the participating hospital and physicians to make decisions about the governance and management of the entity, the criteria for selecting physician members, and the rules for sharing financial risk and profits.

Increased Accountability for Governing Boards

We are now firmly into a third era for hospital governing boards, one characterized by increased emphasis on the accountability of boards for hospital operations, which carries over to the activities of the medical staff. Although fiduciary duties for hospital board members are well established, hospital boards have faced relatively little oversight of their activities.[16] However, this appears to be changing as several developments are bringing hospital boards under much greater scrutiny. For instance, federal agencies responsible for monitoring hospitals are becoming more exacting in their expectations that hospital boards will ensure compliance with the rules and regulations of federal health care reimbursement programs.[17] Because hospital compliance with such rules and regulations depends substantially on the actions of medical staff members, hospital boards must take steps to educate and oversee their medical staffs with respect to issues such as false claims, kickbacks, and prohibitions on self-referral (see Chapter Six).

Increased board accountability for medical staff activities also emanates from the growing demands for measuring and evaluating quality of care.[18] Many public and private payers now collect data pertaining to the quality of care of the health care providers with which hospitals do business. These data may be reported publicly to inform the insured community about providers' relative performance on selected quality measures. Payers are also linking reimbursement to quality performance so that hospital boards have a financial incentive to monitor and, if necessary, remediate the care provided by their medical staff.

Further, there is a trend at the federal and state levels to strengthen hospital governance by imposing requirements on hospital boards in terms of their structure and practices.[19] This development follows a series of corporate scandals that have been attributed in part to weak corporate governance. These scandals occurred during the last decade, chiefly among publicly held companies such as Enron but also including some nonprofits as well (for example, the Allegheny Health Education and Research Foundation). One congressional response to these scandals was the enactment of the landmark legislation popularly known as the Sarbanes-Oxley Act that requires certain board structures and practices for publicly held corporations. Although Sarbanes-Oxley does not apply to nonprofit corporations, the legislation has been an impetus to policymakers to consider whether nonprofits should be subject to similar types of governance requirements.

In general, these initiatives, some of which are designed to closely follow provisions in the Sarbanes-Oxley legislation, seek to accomplish one or more of three objectives: enhance the independence of hospital governing boards, increase board accountability to communities and other key stakeholders, and reduce conflicts of financial interest between board members and the organizations they govern. For example, New Hampshire passed legislation that requires hospitals to obtain community input as part of their process for determining community needs.[20] At the federal level, the Internal Revenue Service (IRS), which is responsible for determining whether nonprofit hospitals qualify for federal income tax exemptions, has announced that it will step up its monitoring of tax-exempt hospitals, including closer examination of these organizations' governance arrangements.[21] Although none of these initiatives directly relates to the board's oversight of the medical staff, they indirectly affect hospital–medical staff relationships by elevating the accountability of the board for the entire hospital enterprise and thus, by implication, casting the medical staff in a somewhat subordinate relationship relative to the board.

Medical Staff Governance

The previous section described how developments in hospital regulation, reimbursement, and competition have eroded the "separate but parallel" basis for alignment between hospitals and physicians in the late twentieth and early twenty-first centuries. However, organizational structure and financial incentives challenge the ability of both hospital governing boards and medical staffs to respond to these pressures. From the perspective of the medical staff, frustration has grown with regard to the ability of medical staff members to influence hospital practice and policy. This has created increasing schisms and mistrust between hospitals and their medical staff and has eroded the basis for aligning the interests of the two parties for purposes of improving quality and reducing costs. Indeed, a major impasse for hospital-physician alignment has been the attitude of many medical staffs that they serve as the last line of defense against poor quality of care, given the growing cost-containment pressures that hospitals face in the era of prospective payment and managed care. This attitude reinforces the perspective that quality of care stems from the individual physician's relationship with the individual patient and that attempts to standardize care processes should be resisted.

Aside from such fundamental differences in orientation to quality and related mistrust over motives and goals, many of the problems of alignment can be traced to medical staff governance itself. In contrast to hospitals, which are organized and governed along bureaucratic lines with clearly established lines of authority and accountability, the members of the typical hospital medical staff are organized as an association of physicians with ties to the hospital but with little else to bind them together as a collective entity. These associations are essentially membership organizations that lack formal authority to impose accountability standards on their members or to direct integrated activity with hospitals.[22] Because of its loose structure and emphasis on individual physician interests, the association form of medical staff governance is not well suited to promoting collective responsibility for patient care quality, operational efficiency, or other areas of performance. Some have argued that the association form of medical staff governance creates a situation where physician leaders perceive an accountability pathway that leads downward toward their members rather than upward toward the hospital board, where legal authority resides. The practical result is that many physician leaders commonly perceive that their charge is to represent the medical staff agenda to the board, rather than to be accountable to the board for quality of care or reducing costs in the institution, as accreditation and legal standards dictate.

Unfortunately, this has led to a situation where medical staff leaders cannot render decisions on important policy or organizational matters without the express consent of those who elected them. Without virtually 100 percent endorsement from their colleagues, their action can be inordinately slow and consensus can be difficult to achieve around key policy or strategic issues. Although it might appear dysfunctional, this rather cumbersome governance structure is consistent with the fundamental value position of most physicians that ensuring quality is an individual, professional responsibility, not a collective one. This individualistic orientation further erodes power and cohesion of the medical staff, and some have even, half jokingly, observed that the medical staff organization is an organization in name only.

Although one could argue that strong leadership in the hospital medical staff could overcome both the structural barriers to alignment (for example, the association form of medical staffs) and the fragmented voice of physicians on the medical staff (for example, primary care versus specialists), the leadership of medical staffs is often insufficiently prepared or trained to overcome these barriers. Further, the last several years have witnessed less physician involvement with hospital and medical staff affairs, as office-based practice and nonhospital procedures assume a greater share of physician business.[23] This has led to weak leadership and uninvolved membership as well as competitive tensions between hospitals and their own medical staffs. Thus there is a growing tendency for physicians to view their medical staff organization obligations with some degree of disdain. These obligations are typically perceived as bureaucratic busywork required chiefly to fulfill the needs of a questionably legitimate source of accountability.

Although many physicians understand and accept a responsibility to advise administration and to maintain licensure and accreditation, they often perceive time consumed by organizational activities as being of little relevance to their hospital practices. As a derivative of the hospital-as-workshop model, physicians often tend to equate what is good for the community with what they perceive as supportive of their medical practice. Board members, in contrast, correctly see their fundamental role as overseers of public trust. They might be incompletely aware that many physicians view the board's primary responsibility to the community as one of ensuring resources with which physicians can optimally practice their professions. These fundamentally different perceptions of the community hospital and its role can be a source of major misunderstanding and potential conflict between the hospital and medical staff.

The need to work around the largely ungovernable traditional hospital medical staffs and their lack of clear collective accountability has given rise to the previously discussed organizational arrangements designed to selectively partner physicians and hospitals to advance particular clinical and strategic interests. These work-around structures, including joint ventures, PHOs, MSOs, and other specialized clinical endeavors, are often jointly sponsored by the organized medical staff leadership and hospital management. They are often focused on particular conditions or clinical service lines and involve selected (or self-selected) members of the medical staff and relevant members of the hospital management team.[24] The board's oversight responsibility for these structures remains unclear, particularly because these arrangements often are affiliates or subsidiaries, rather than clinical units, of the hospital. In other words, it is not completely clear *what* is being governed. For example, should there be a direct line of authority between the governance structures of these new entities and the board of the hospital? Do governing board members have the obligation to serve on the governing bodies of the new entities? Do new structures fall outside the legal boundaries that define traditional hospital medical staff relationships?

In sum, the traditional hospital medical staff leadership appears to be ill equipped to assume collective responsibility for quality and cost reduction in the delivery of patient care and to be a partner with the hospital board. It is a structure designed to enhance the economic position and clinical prerogatives of individual physicians and not collective responsibility for ensuring that populations of patients receive high-quality care. Hospital boards' abrogation of oversight responsibility over medical staff activities further reinforces the disconnect between these two groups. Whereas the medical staff is formally and legally accountable to the board of the hospital, in practice this accountability is rarely exercised in a way that would strengthen the collective effort to ensure high-quality and efficient care. Problems that have led to this situation are both structural and cultural. Neither the association structure nor the fragmented composition of the medical staff lends itself to increased accountability. Finally, differences between the cultural orientation of physicians to individual patient care and the collective orientation of hospital boards to the community and to a population of patients have made common ground difficult to achieve.

Additional Challenges to Governance and Alignment

Although the basic governance structure of the hospital and medical staff has remained largely unchanged in the last fifty years, relationships between hospitals and medical staffs have undergone significant changes. There have been increased demands for board accountability for hospital activities that are deeply affected by the behavior of medical staff members.[25] This raises questions as to the ability of hospital boards to fully discharge their governance responsibilities in ways that will secure the necessary cooperation of the medical staff, given the medical staff's limited self-governance. What is the potential for the hospital board to realign the interests of the hospital and the medical staff in a way that ensures the viability of the hospital and effectively discharges its governance responsibilities for both the institution's financial and clinical performance? In fact, there are numerous barriers and challenges for the board to be effective in this role, some of which are internal and some of which are external to the hospital.

Internal Challenges

One of the foremost internal challenges to better hospital-physician alignment is the unique situation of physicians in most hospitals as quasi-independent practitioners. As discussed earlier in this chapter, this situation creates problems of diffuse authority and unstable spheres of influence among the medical staff, the management, and the governing body. This contrasts markedly with a typical business corporation in which the board exercises direct control over the corporate CEO, who in turn has full authority over the operations of the corporation, including its personnel. Yet, as noted, physicians assign a very high value to their professional autonomy and ability to function outside the bureaucratic controls of the hospital, and boards lack adequate mechanisms to hold medical staff members accountable for their performance, even though the board is in effect accountable for that performance.

At the same time, however, hospital employment of physicians is unlikely to be a silver bullet solution to this internal challenge. Hospital acquisition of physician practices was common during the 1990s, as many hospital executives believed that an employment model was necessary for securing the control over physicians that hospitals needed to adapt successfully to managed care and reimbursement pressures. However, many hospitals experienced significant financial disappointments with these acquisitions.[26] Although several factors contributed to these disappointing financial results, it also became apparent that employment of physicians did not guarantee their loyalty and cooperation relative to the hospital and its goals. Survey results from one large study indicated that although employed physicians reported on average a higher level of commitment to the hospital than those who were not employed, the difference was quite small, suggesting that structural arrangements by themselves are not sufficient for strengthening hospital-physician alignment.[27]

The financial meltdown of the once formidable Allegheny Health Care System is also instructive on this point as an example of health care system governance gone wrong despite the use of physician employment and other structural arrangements that were widely considered to be progressive at the time.[28] The Allegheny situation is particularly important because it emphasizes that even tight integration between hospital and physicians (for example, physician employment) did not necessarily result in alignment or better quality care. Fundamental to Allegheny's problems were discrepancies in decision making between the system and its member hospitals through the governing boards—which were central decision-making bodies with control over the entire system—and lack of comparable, unified governance among physician groups affiliated with the system. As a result, physicians typically remained fragmented in their objectives, and their interests localized. Such problems were often exaggerated by differences among physicians themselves (for example, specialist versus primary care physicians, academic versus community physicians, employed physicians versus independent contractors). The bottom line for Allegheny was that despite an ostensibly centralized and integrated organization, lack of collaborative governance and disorganized governance for the medical staff led to inefficiencies, conflict, and unrealized organizational goals.[29]

A second internal challenge to stronger hospital-physician alignment is board members' lack of health care background or clinical expertise. Board members are often selected on the basis of their business experience, professional skills (legal, marketing, finance), community ties, personal values, and time availability.[30] Although board members from manufacturing and service industries may be well versed in quality issues, board members report feeling confused about their responsibility for quality of care, ill prepared to evaluate quality of care, and uncomfortable taking action to rectify a quality problem (for example, denying physician reappointment or disciplining an incompetent physician).[31] The previously noted trend toward inclusion of medical staff members on hospital boards may be helping to alleviate this problem to some degree. There is also evidence that boards are more engaged today than in the past in reviewing quality-related clinical data.[32] Nevertheless, boards continue to be challenged in meeting their responsibilities to oversee the clinical activities of the medical staff, even though this oversight has a direct bearing on the hospital's overall efficiency and quality of care.

External Challenges

External to the hospital, numerous legal and regulatory policies serve as barriers to tighter integration between hospital and medical staff. All of these laws and regulations are discussed in greater detail in Chapter Six.

As noted, many states have long had in place a policy that prohibits corporations from employing physicians directly—the so-called corporate practice of medicine doctrine—which serves to reinforce the legitimacy of the voluntary medical staff with its previously noted difficulties. However, even in states such as California that rigorously enforce this policy, the prohibition itself is fairly easy to circumvent through professional service agreements that substitute for employment relationships but accomplish much the same goals. Many of the states that have the policy also provide certain exceptions, such as for teaching hospitals.[33] More substantial legal and regulatory barriers come in the form of fraud and abuse provisions, namely the federal antikickback statute and the Stark laws on self-referral. These provisions are intended to limit the role of financial incentives in provider referral decisions for clinical services. However, because these provisions are broad and somewhat vague in their language, the scope of their application is extensive in deterring hospitals and physicians from engaging in legitimate business collaborations that are mutually beneficial and potentially promote patient care. As a result, hospitals and physicians need to proceed cautiously in forming joint ventures and engaging in gainsharing to improve quality and efficiency.

Federal and state antitrust laws—and fear about them—also sometimes stand in the way of greater hospital-medical staff collaboration. Antitrust enforcement authorities raise concerns about arrangements whereby hospitals are potentially in a position to facilitate price collusion among medical staff members who are otherwise competitors in the practice of medicine. For example, physician hospital organizations and management service organizations are both vehicles for collaboration between hospital and medical staff but also vehicles that can arouse suspicion on the part of antitrust enforcement authorities. Further, as most nonprofit hospitals are exempt from federal income tax, the IRS also has a say in whether and how hospitals and medical staff collaborate. Many of the collaborative arrangements that present potential fraud and abuse concerns also potentially put in jeopardy a hospital's tax-exempt status, especially if the arrangement is seen as violating the prohibition on private benefit or inurement, whereby tax-exempt entities are not allowed to distribute any income in the form of dividends to any person.

Accordingly, hospitals and physicians undoubtedly find themselves between a rock and a hard place as heightened competitive pressures and changing reimbursement systems call for greater integration, but various legal and regulatory provisions sharply limit the range of collaborative ventures that are possible. The inherent difficulty of working out more collaborative relationships between physicians and health systems is made more difficult when the external policy environment creates conflicting incentives and mixed signals regarding the desirability of vertical integration.[34]

The Board of the Future: Moving Beyond Oversight to Collaborative Leadership

In spite of the myriad problems that have precluded hospital governing boards and medical staffs from developing collaborations that would better align the hospital and its physicians, there are some signs of hope in this area. The previously noted policy developments that expand hospital boards' accountability for hospital quality, for example, have made board oversight over medical staff activities and admitting privileges more salient. Hospital boards can no longer discharge their responsibilities for quality by delegating quality matters to the medical staff and thereafter assuming that all will be well. Similarly, government initiatives to ensure that hospitals meet their obligations for maintaining tax-exempt status have also sensitized boards to the importance of gaining the cooperation of the hospital's medical staff.[35]

In this context, hospital board members are often placed in the position of mediating between conflicting interests of physicians and administrators as both respond to changing market demands imposed by managed care firms, large employers, and a changing regulatory and tax environment. This suggests that the primary role of hospital boards in the future will be to clearly communicate a vision for the organization and to ensure that all parties (internal and external) engage in strategies to achieve that vision. Put another way, the focus of governance in hospitals is migrating beyond compliance and oversight toward strategic and collaborative leadership. Indeed, the board is the only structural interface through which elements of leadership in the community, management, and the medical staff can jointly establish, communicate, and evaluate a common vision for improved quality in the hospital. The board provides an important link between strategy or mission and the allocation of resources, such as revising management and physicians' compensation and incentives to ensure that the broader vision and goals of the institution are achieved. There are several specific leverage points under the board's control that can be used to strengthen alignment between hospitals and physicians. These leverage points are establishing a leadership role for the board in quality of care; improving styles of communication within the organization; changing perceptions of medical professionalism; and extending a spirit of collaboration to the new joint ventures (or work-arounds) that hospitals and physicians have begun to create as a means of achieving common goals.

Leadership for Quality

Quality improvement is likely to serve as the most powerful impetus for governance reform. Hospital boards must come to grips with their responsibility for ensuring the quality of care provided in the institutions they govern. This responsibility for quality has been well established by numerous legal precedents, but as previously noted, many boards have yet to fully understand, much less actively engage in discharging, this responsibility.[36] Boards can play a leadership role by establishing quality and patient safety as organizational priorities, allocating resources to support quality improvement efforts, and revising executive compensation and performance to emphasize quality of care. Boards are also in a position to spearhead a shift toward a culture of patient safety and high quality in their institutions.

These quality-related priorities should be embraced by hospital management but should particularly resonate with physicians who share similar values. Making quality a priority with the attendant allocation of resources and emphasis on clinical improvement will have the effect of engaging physicians at a high level. If the board is to emphasize quality improvement, it must incorporate extensive clinical input. This may suggest that boards increase alignment with their physicians by including more physicians, nurses, and other clinicians among their members.

Although physician membership on hospital boards has been advocated in the past, it has rarely been done with the intention of reinforcing hospitals' strategic emphasis on improved quality and patient safety. What must be avoided is including individuals who represent medical staff interests and not organizational interests more broadly. This may require the board to review and possibly amend bylaws to ensure that physician board service extends beyond an ex officio representative of medical staff with a permanent seat on the hospital board.

From a slightly different perspective, the traditional hands-off posture of hospital board members toward the medical staff must be changed to allow board members to take a more active role in medical staff affairs. This might take the form of having board members sit on medical staff committees, particularly those that discuss strategies for improving quality of care and patient safety. Although such strategies will improve the level of communication between the hospital and medical staff, they may carry some risk of being perceived as threatening to physician autonomy and self-governance. To ensure these strategies are successful, hospital trustees should therefore take pains to reassert their legal obligation for fiduciary oversight of the medical staff. This might include review and revision of hospital and medical staff bylaws to emphasize greater correspondence between hospital and medical staff functions and structures, and to introduce accountability standards. Tactically, revisions to hospital medical staff bylaws should be done through a joint conference committee of physicians and board members. This may blunt threats to physician autonomy and self-governance and ensure that changes in bylaws are realistic and not seen as top-down control over physician affairs.

In order for hospital board members to effectively exercise their quality oversight responsibility over medical staff affiliated with the hospital, better information about physician outcomes and clinical quality must be available to them. Often, quality information is too technical or too clinical for board members to understand and appreciate. This exacerbates the tendency to defer completely to clinical members of the board or to delegate responsibility for quality to the hospital medical staff without appropriate oversight. Further, because hospital quality and outcomes have been so poorly measured, there has been little incentive for boards to exercise oversight beyond that minimally required to reduce liability exposure or avoid jeopardizing accreditation.

Saint John's clinic in Southwest Missouri is an example of a health care system that revised its governance structure to improve leadership around quality (and cost) issues. Saint John's accomplished this by creating a physician governing body on an equal level with the hospital to promote fundamental, operational changes and to develop a unified culture upon which an integrated health care system could be built. The goal of this dual, or equal, governance structure was to create an organization that would allow for greater physician authority and accountability in the management of physician practices and to develop a sustainable future financial model for the clinic. This took the form of creating separate clinical governance in individual physician's business units and at the same time integrating the physician practices as co-equal corporations into the health care system.

The heart of these governance arrangements was the building of a collaborative relationship between the governing boards and management by fostering qualified, knowledgeable physician boards that actively engaged in policymaking and strategy making in coordination with the hospital board. The hospital also allocated resources to help medical practices increase organizational efficiency and effectiveness by linking information technology. On the medical staff side, physician governing boards increased their effort to communicate with their staff colleagues through constructive two-way communications, shared learning, and a nonthreatening style of engagement. Finally, in the important area of resource allocations, distribution of resources was done formally on the basis of constructed business plans by physician and administrative teams.[37]

Improving Communications

Any governance-based approach to increase alignment between hospitals and physicians must enhance the type and scope of communications between boards and medical staff. As noted previously, hospital boards typically relate to medical staffs primarily in terms of delegating responsibility for physician credentialing to medical staff leadership. However, communications between board and medical staff often do not extend to issues related to strategy and other major initiatives undertaken by a hospital that could directly or indirectly affect its physicians. Although it is important to recognize that medical staffs themselves have contributed to this lack of two-way communication, by invoking autonomy and self-governance, efforts can be made to overcome these historical patterns to establish a foundation for collaboration.

In regard to content of communication, hospital boards need to be especially conscious of decisions in areas that on the surface may not strike them as relevant to physicians but that often have direct implications for clinical practice. These include issues related to strategic planning, manpower planning, budgeting, and capital expenditures, all of which may carry implications for change in the clinical culture of the hospital.

Redefining Medical Professionalism

The board can also take a leading role in shaping and communicating how principles of medical professionalism must change in order to address responsibilities of clinicians, not only to individual patients but also to the organization, its mission, and its governing board. This type of cultural transformation will require strong leadership on both the medical staff side and the hospital board. A notable example of revised accountability in clinical governance is the Kaiser Permanente system in California. Besides recruiting doctors who believe in keeping patients healthy, Kaiser is organized so that all doctors from primary, secondary, and tertiary care share budget responsibility for all care. This arrangement has required generalists and specialists to resolve their long-standing differences to determine ways to minimize costly hospital services and maximize cost effectiveness. In contrast, many hospitals and health care systems still give little attention to the physician role in organizational governance. As noted, physician participation in governance is often limited to a physician or two on the hospital board, a chief medical officer serving on governance committees, and physicians serving as chairs of clinical departments.

Work-Arounds

Hospital boards seeking to strengthen alignment with physicians often face a strategic choice. On one hand, they may focus on joint representation on hospital and medical staff governing committees and improving hospital culture so physicians can view the organization as advancing their interests and values. Alternately (or perhaps simultaneously), boards can try to work around the hospital medical staff by creating a parallel set of structures and activities such as physician hospital organizations, foundations, and joint ventures that select willing members of the medical staff and those whose interests and priorities align with those of the hospital.

When pursuing the latter strategy, board members must be cognizant of ventures that hospitals and physicians are undertaking to align their interests outside the formal structure of the hospital and medical staff. Although these arrangements provide flexibility for aligning hospital and physician activity, board members must oversee them to ensure that they are consistent with the hospital's mission and do not divert resources, present conflicts of interest, or diminish the hospital's basic purpose.

Organizational forms such as physician hospital organizations, foundations, and medical service organizations, originally established to improve the position of the hospital for managed care contracting, can be reinvented to focus on issues of improving quality of care, patient safety, and forming strategic partnerships that represent greater alignment between the hospital and its medical staff. The key to making such structures effective is working out a system of joint governance that coordinates decision making and provides adequate representation of both clinical and hospital interests.

It is important to understand that alternative approaches to hospital and medical staff collaboration will succeed only if hospital governing boards and executive management are prepared to cede real power to physicians. This means that physician power needs to be organized and exercised to improve quality and reduce costs, rather than being held by a few prominent or assertive physicians and exercised arbitrarily, as has often been the case in the past. Indeed, one of the inherent but often unstated assumptions of these alternative arrangements is the notion that physicians would take substantial ownership, as well as accountability, for the patient care services provided in these arrangements. This suggests that boards of hospitals must exercise sufficient oversight in understanding the purpose of these arrangements and their relationship to hospital strategy and mission but yield control and discretion to physician participants as far as operations. Governing bodies therefore must strike a sensitive balance between respecting medical groups' control over medical practice, quality assurance, and quality improvement activities, while also ensuring that the hospital's mission and goals are not diverted or undermined by activities of these subsidiary organizations. Often this means that boards must draft very specific documentation outlining roles and expectations of both parties, and sometimes make allowances for competition with physicians in some areas while engaging in collaboration with the same physicians in others.

In many respects, the presence of these work-around organizations adds complexity to the governance system of hospitals. At the same time, it affords a more flexible approach to pursuing joint strategic interests than trying to work with the hospital medical staff directly. However, it would be disingenuous to suggest that structural arrangements created to align physician and hospital interests are universally effective in accomplishing these goals. Previous research suggests that hospital-physician arrangements are often only loosely coupled to strategies and processes used to govern them.[38]

Governance is the glue that binds these structures together and makes them potentially effective as strategic vehicles for aligning hospital and physicians' interests. For example, the foundation model typically takes the form of a corporation, usually nonprofit, that is organized either as an affiliate of the hospital with a common parent organization or as a subsidiary of a hospital. The foundation owns and operates one or more practices, including practice facilities, equipment, and supplies. The foundation also employs all the nonphysician personnel and contracts with the physician-owned entity to provide medical services for the practice. A foundation is governed by a combination of representatives from the physician group, the hospital, and the community. Physician representation in foundation governance is limited by the Internal Revenue Service to no more than 49 percent of practitioners in the medical group (due to IRS reluctance to exempt physician-controlled entities from taxation). Indeed a majority of these boards' members are required by the IRS to be nonpaid community leaders or nonphysician hospital representatives.[39] The fact that the foundation board comprises a large segment of the affiliated physician group as well as other relevant stakeholders makes it an attractive governance structure for the specific goals of the entity.

Unlike the hospital, which is typically subject to multiple missions and objectives, the foundation model or other physician organization arrangement can be more specialized in its purpose and thus can draw on a self-selected group of executives and physicians for its governance. This makes it more likely that there will be fewer conflicts and that the various stakeholders involved will be able to come to common agreement on policies and operating practices. The keys to governance success in these models are legal separation from the complex hospital regulatory and reimbursement environment, a self-selected group of physicians who presumably share interests with the foundation goals, and a vehicle for representing the interests and objectives of the hospital through membership on the foundation board.

Conclusion

As this chapter goes to press, a major health care reform initiative is undergoing debate in Congress, an initiative that could potentially lead to fundamental changes in the organization of the health care industry in the United States.

Whatever reform initiatives do come to pass, several actions need to be undertaken to enable hospital governing boards to effectively align hospitals and physicians for the purpose of improving the delivery of health care services. It is important to realize that because governance issues are systemic, it is unlikely that any one of these changes will have the desired effect on alignment without acting on other issues. The following recommendations focus on simultaneously addressing changes to both hospital and medical staff governance and the payment and regulatory contexts in which these entities operate:

1. **Payers should reform reimbursement policies to establish common financial incentives for hospitals and physicians**. As noted elsewhere in this book, payment systems for hospital and physician services have played an important role in shaping the nature of the hospital-physician relationship in the United States. Although payment systems enabled hospitals and physicians to peacefully coexist throughout much of the twentieth century, these systems did not encourage either party to closely coordinate with the other in terms of patient care. More recently, payment systems have sometimes placed hospitals and physicians in an adversarial position. Thus, for hospital boards to be more effective in aligning hospitals and physicians, payment systems need to be changed to create financial incentives for hospitals and physicians to work collaboratively. Some progress has already been made on this front as payers have experimented with episode-based payments to hospitals and physicians for co-managing patient care with respect to particular procedures or episodes. Capitation or global payments also may be used to create financial incentives for strengthening hospital-physician alignment. These types of payment arrangements have not yet been implemented on a wide-scale basis. Accordingly, payers need to expand their efforts in this direction so that board members and medical staff have a financial incentive for working together to improve patient care.

2. **Hospital boards should undergo training to strengthen capabilities around managing the hospital-physician interface**. To meet the challenges that have been identified for hospital governance, hospital boards need to first engage in careful self-assessment of their own development and orientation relative to their responsibilities. As noted, many board members lack the experience and skills to effectively carry out the activities necessary to strengthen hospital-physician alignment. Hospitals require board members with the skills for overseeing quality of care. They also need board members who understand the cultural barriers that separate hospital management from physicians and who can take the steps to help close those barriers through the development

and communication of a common vision and related strategies. Rather than the traditional hands-off posture taken by many boards, successful boards need members who are able to reach out to medical staff members and cultivate a culture that embraces them within an organizational framework that does not rely exclusively on structural arrangements for aligning them with the hospital.

3. **Medical staff governance should shift from a representative or association orientation to one of collective accountability**. In concert with changes in the hospital board outlined earlier, hospital medical staffs must undertake fundamental cultural, leadership, and organizational changes aimed at increasing *collective*, not just *individual*, accountability for both quality and costs in the hospital. Operationally, this may entail shifting the dominant focus of medical staff governance away from ensuring individual, clinical expertise of its members and advancing physician interests exclusively. Instead, emphasis should be placed on developing greater collaborative governance arrangements with the hospital board, strengthening leadership and leadership development in medical staffs to make such positions more effective, attractive, and meaningful to physicians, and revising medical staff charters and bylaws to formally reflect collective responsibility for quality and costs in hospitals. Perhaps most fundamentally, the culture of medical staff governance needs to shift from a representative model whereby individual or subgroup interests are paramount and accountability flows downward, to a governance model that emphasizes collective responsibility for patient care and promotes the mutual interests of hospitals and physicians.

4. **Policymakers should review and selectively revise pertinent legal and regulatory provisions**. Policymakers should review and, where appropriate, modify legal and regulatory provisions that impede effective hospital-physician collaboration. This is not a call for massive legal reform but rather for a detailed review of the legal and regulatory structures that currently relate to hospital-physician relationships to sort out what provisions continue to serve legitimate objectives and what provisions have become largely barriers with little if any offsetting benefits. As noted, current legal and regulatory structures have created conflicting incentives around hospital-physician collaborations that are difficult if not impossible to reconcile. Accordingly, hospital boards need to be liberated from some of the legal and regulatory provisions that impede their ability to align hospitals and physicians. Legal restrictions on gainsharing arrangements between hospitals and physicians are a particularly controversial example, but other legal and regulatory provisions are also in need of evaluation, including those pertaining to antitrust, fraud and abuse, and tax exemption.

Notes

1. L. Shi and D. Singh, *Essentials of the U.S. Healthcare System* (Sudbury, MA: Jones & Bartlett, 2010).
2. N. Ono, "Boards of Directors Under Fire: An Examination of Nonprofit Board Duties in the Health Care Environment," *Annals of Health Law* 7 (1998): 107–38.
3. T. Alexander, and L. Weaver, "Roles and Responsibilities of Community Nonprofit Boards," *Nonprofit Management and Leadership* 10, no. 2 (2003): 153–67.
4. J. R. Griffith and K. R. White, *The Well-Managed Healthcare Organization*, 5th ed. (Chicago: Health Administration Press, 2002).
5. J. A. Alexander and T. L. Amburgey, "The Dynamics of Change in the American Hospital Industry: Transformation or Selection," *Medical Care Review* 44 (1987): 279–321; J. A. Alexander, "Hospital Trusteeship in an Era of Institutional Transition: What Can We Learn from Governance Research?" in *The Ethics of Hospital Trustees*, ed. B. Jennings and B. Gray, 1–15 (Washington, D.C.: Georgetown University Press, 2004).
6. P. M. Starr, *The Social Transformation of American Medicine* (New York: Basic Books, 1982); Alexander and Amburgey. "The Dynamics of Change in the American Hospital Industry."
7. J. A. Alexander and H. Zuckerman, "Health Care Governance: Are We Keeping Pace?" *Journal of Health Administration Education* 7, no. 4 (1989): 760–77; Starr, *Social Transformation of American Medicine*.
8. B. J. Weiner and J. A. Alexander, "Corporate and Philanthropic Models of Hospital Governance: A Taxonomic Evaluation," *Health Services Research* 28 (1993): 325–55.
9. L. R. Burns, R. M. Andersen, and S. M. Shortell, "The Effect of Hospital Control Strategies on Physician Satisfaction and Hospital-Physician Conflict," *Health Services Research* 25 (1990): 527–60; E. Simendinger and W. Pasmore, "Developing Partnerships Between Physicians and Healthcare Executives," *Hospital and Health Services Administration* 29, no. 6 (November/December 1984): 21–35; S. M. Shortell, *Effective Hospital-Physician Relationships* (Ann Arbor, MI: Health Administration Press, 1991).
10. J. Zwanziger and G. A. Melnick, "Effects of Competition on the Hospital Industry: Evidence from California," in *Competitive Approaches to Health Care Reform*, ed. R. Arnould, R. Rich, and W. White, 111–138 (Washington, D.C.: Urban Institute Press, 1992); G. Young, J. Burgess, and D. Valley, "Competition Among Hospitals for the Business of HMOs: Effect of Price and Non-Price Attributes," *Health Services Research* 37 (2002): 1267–90.
11. American Hospital Association, *Status of Capital Control Expenditure Programs* (Chicago: American Hospital Association, 1987).
12. J. A. Alexander, L. L. Morlock, and B. Gifford, "The Effects of Corporate Restructuring on Hospital Policymaking," *Health Services Research* 23 (1988): 311–38; G. Young, "Insider Representation on the Governing Boards of Nonprofit Hospitals: Trends and Implications for Charitable Care," *Inquiry* 33 (1997): 352–62.
13. Young, "Insider Representation."
14. C. Molinari, L. Morlock, J. Alexander, and C. A. Lyles, "Hospital Board Effectiveness: Relationships Between Governing Board Composition and Hospital Financial Viability," *Health Services Research* 28 (1993): 269–92; C. Molinari, L. Morlock, J. Alexander, and C. A. Lyles, "Does the Hospital Board Need a Doctor?" *Medical Care* 33 (1995): 170–85; Young, "Insider Representation."

15. L. R. Burns and D. P. Thorpe, "Trends and Models in Physician-Hospital Organizations," *Health Care Management Review* 18 (1993): 7–20.

16. J. R. Schwartz and H. C. Horn, *Health Care Alliances and Conversions: A Handbook for Nonprofit Trustees* (San Francisco: Jossey-Bass, 1999).

17. Office of Inspector General (OIG), U.S. Department of Health and Human Services, and American Health Lawyers Association, *Corporate Responsibility and Corporate Compliance: A Resource for Health Care Boards of Directors* (2003). http://oig.hhs.gov/fraud/docs/complianceguidannce/040203corpresprsceguide.pdf.

18. Weiner and Alexander, "Corporate and Philanthropic Models of Hospital Governance."

19. J. Alexander, G. Young, B. Weiner, and L. Hearld, "Governance and Community Benefit: Are Nonprofit Hospitals Good Candidates for Sarbanes-Oxley Reforms?" *Journal of Health Politics, Policy and Law* 33 (2008): 199–224.

20. PriceWaterhouseCoopers, "Sarbanes-Oxley Update," Health Research Institute (Not-for-Profit Healthcare Update, May 2005 [second in series]). www.pwc.com/extweb/pwcpublications.nsf/docid/9A2A5DCCB20B390B525700E0064DEEF.

21. J. E. Orlikoff, "Building Better Boards in the New Era of Accountability," *Frontiers of Health Services Management* 21, no. 3 (2005): 3–12.

22. A. Gosfield, "The Organized Medical Staff: Should Anyone Care Anymore?" *Medical Practice Management*, January/February 2005: 210–16.

23. Gosfield, "The Organized Medical Staff."

24. T. Lake, K. Devers, L. Brewster, and L. Casalino, "Something Old, Something New: Recent Developments in Hospital-Physician Relationships," *Health Services Research* 38, no. 1 (2003): 471–87; L. R. Burns and D. R. Wholey, "Responding to a Consolidating Healthcare System: Options for Physician Organizations," *Future of Integrated Delivery Systems* 1 (2000): 261–323.

25. J. A. Alexander, B. Weiner, and R. Bogue, "Changes in the Structure, Composition, and Activity of Hospital Governing Boards 1989–1997: Evidence from Two National Surveys,"*Milbank Quarterly* 79 (2001): 253–79.

26. Cain Brothers [investment bankers and capital advisers], "Going, Going, Gone . . . Physician Disassociation: A Home Run?"*Strategies in Capital Finance* 31 (Summer 2000).

27. L. R. Burns, S. L. Walston, J. A. Alexander, H. S. Zuckerman, and others, "Just How Integrated Are Integrated Delivery Systems? Results from a National Survey," *Health Care Management Review* 26, no. 1 (2001): 22–41.

28. Burns and Wholey, "Responding to a Consolidating Healthcare System."

29. L. R. Burns, J. Cacciamani, J. Clement, and W. Aquino, "The Fall of the House of AHERF: The Allegheny Bankruptcy," *Health Affairs* 19, no. 1 (2000): 7–41.

30. K. Gautam and J. Goodstein, "Insiders and Business Directors on Hospital Boards and Strategic Change,"*Hospital and Health Services Administration* 41 (1996): 423–40.

31. B. J. Weiner and J. A. Alexander, "Corporate and Philanthropic Models of Hospital Governance: A Taxonomic Evaluation," *Health Services Research* 28 (1993): 325–55.

32. Alexander, Weiner, and Bogue, "Changes in the Structure, Composition, and Activity of Hospital Governing Boards 1989–1997."

33. L. R. Burns and D. P. Thorpe, "Trends and Models in Physician-Hospital Organizations."

34. Burns and Wholey, "Responding to a Consolidating Healthcare System."

35. Orlikoff, "Building Better Boards in the New Era of Accountability."

36. A. K. Jha and A. M. Epstein, "Hospital Governance and the Quality of Care," *Health Affairs* Web exclusive (November 6, 2009) http://content.healthaffairs.org/cgi/content/abstract/hlthaff.2009.0297.

37. M. Goler and D. Sorensen, "Physician Governance—The Strength Behind St. John's Clinic," *Physician Executive* (January/February, 2006), 1–9.
38. J. A. Alexander, L. Burns, H. Zuckerman, T. Vaughn, and others, "An Exploratory Analysis of Market-Based Physician-Organization Arrangements," *Hospital and Health Services Administration* 41, no. 3 (Fall 1996): 311–29.
39. L. R. Burns and D. P. Thorpe, "Trends and Models in Physician-Hospital Organizations."

Commentaries

James A. DeNuccio, Director, Organized Medical Staff Services, American Medical Association

The American Medical Association (AMA), whose mission is to promote the art and science of medicine and the betterment of public health, has extensive policy that provides guidance to physicians and others related to governance, collaboration, and payment. The relationship between the organized medical staff and the governing body varies from organization to organization. The medical staffs and governing bodies of individual hospitals are positioned at different points on the described continuum.

Physicians, hospital governing bodies, and senior managers as their representatives have a mutual responsibility to cooperate in effectively maintaining patient care. Strengthening a hospital's alignment with the active practicing physician will improve the quality, efficiency, and accessibility of care. In the hospital setting, realization of these benefits can be facilitated through a more collaborative relationship.

The organized medical staff and its members have a contractual obligation, entered into with the hospital, to carry out their professional medical responsibilities and to function as a self-governing body to promote quality patient care within the hospital. The organized medical staff and its members are responsible for and accountable to the governing body for the quality of care provided to patients by the hospital.

Ongoing, timely, and effective communication by and between the hospital governing body and the organized medical staff is critical to a constructive working relationship. The organized medical staff has inherent rights of self-governance. In addition, the organized medical staff should elect appropriate member representation to attend hospital governing body meetings with rights of voice and vote, to ensure appropriate input into hospital governance. Individual members of the organized medical staff should be eligible for full membership on the hospital governing body. Unfortunately, hospital organizations and their governing bodies are not always structured in a manner that encourages and invites this involvement. AMA policy H-225.957, "Principles for Strengthening the Physician-Hospital Relationship," provides extensive guidance in support of an effective working relationship. Many of these tenets can serve as guidance for evolving organizations.

As noted, it is the policy of the AMA that individual physicians who are members of the medical staff—as well as other physicians—should be eligible for full membership on hospital governing bodies and their action committees. Furthermore, the AMA supports medical staff representation on administrative committees of governing bodies and hospital administration representation on administrative committees of the medical staff. Likewise, hospital conflict-of-interest policies for governing board members should apply equally to physician medical staff members of such boards.

Increased physician membership on hospital governing bodies would allow more informed, patient-centered decision making to occur. A governing body must look to and take full advantage of the physician community's medical expertise. Without this involvement, the patients' and the community's needs may not be adequately considered. To foster the necessary involvement, active practicing physicians and their elected leaders must have a consequential role in the decision making of the governing body.

Hospital-associated medical specialists and all members of the medical staff are expected to contribute a reasonable amount of their time, without compensation, to participate in hospital staff committee activities for the purpose of improving patient care, providing continuing education for the benefit of the medical staff, and assisting in the training of physicians and allied health personnel.

Control of community health care services by nonphysicians (laypeople) or with the limited participation of physicians or to the exclusion of other providers in the community may be contrary to the objectives of improving quality and access and providing efficient care. An unintentionally misguided governing body, in the exercise of its fiduciary responsibilities, may misallocate the limited resources available to serve the needs of the community. Increased alignment would facilitate improving care in that hospital but should not occur at the expense of the patient-physician relationship. Creating an entity or relationship that could exclude community physicians from participating or providing care to their patients could be anticompetitive and deprive community physicians and their patients of access to needed services.

The AMA supports the concept of physician governance of health care delivery systems. To meet the broader needs of the community at large, organizations that are independent of hospitals and led by physicians may be in a better position to effectively manage care. These delivery systems should establish self-governing medical staffs similar to those in hospitals. American Medical Association policies

H-285.931, "The Critical Role of Physicians in Health Plans and Integrated Delivery Systems," and H-285.954, "Physician Decision-Making in Health Care Systems," provide extensive guidance to organizations on the physician role in health care delivery systems and highlight the paramount requirements of their involvement.

Concerning reimbursement policies, the AMA is opposed to hospital control of the distribution of any bundled payments to physicians. Further, AMA Code of Medical Ethics Opinion E-8.054, "Financial Incentives and the Practice of Medicine," notes that the size of the patient pool considered in calculations of incentive payments will affect the proximity of financial motivations to individual treatment decisions. Physicians practicing in plans with large numbers of patients in a risk pool therefore have greater freedom to provide the care they feel is necessary based on the likelihood that the needs of other plan patients will balance out decisions to provide extensive care. Consequently, groupings of physicians larger than a single organized medical staff and that staff's patients may better serve quality and cost concerns.

The AMA supports greater physician involvement in hospital governance and encourages collaboration. Without the benefit of physician knowledge of care delivery, patient needs, and their clinical expertise, the ability to improve the delivery and quality of care would be severely limited. Furthermore, the objectives of improving quality, efficiency, and access for the broader community may be better served by independent physician-led organizations that are not exclusionary.

John R. Combes, Senior Vice President, American Hospital Association

With or without health care reform legislation, consumer, clinical, and financial pressures will require greater collaboration between hospitals and health systems and their clinicians, in particular their physicians. The public is demanding more seamless health care, the complexity of care technology and delivery is increasing, and the financial underpinnings of the health care system are unsustainable. Alexander and Young have described well how these forces have shaped the role of health care governance in articulating the vision of its organization and holding the organization accountable for fulfillment of its mission. The board cannot accomplish this role without the support and participation of the medical staff.

While there are many barriers to this level of collaboration, boards—through their diverse perspective and experience—can do much to overcome these obstacles. Boards and physicians have in common the community in which they work and live. By aligning the organization's values with those core professional values of physicians, boards can lessen the level of mutual mistrust between hospitals and their physicians and focus their activities for their community's benefit. As Alexander and Young point out, the clear articulation of the organization's vision and the motivation for all parties to engage in achieving that vision is the primary strategic role of the board. The authors offer several leverage points for boards to use in helping them fulfill that role.

Starting with leadership for quality, boards must be better versed in their role of creating an organizational environment for high quality results. This begins with their focus on mission and extends to their role in assuring the development of an appropriate quality and safety culture, creating the right leadership for the board, management and medical staff, positioning quality and the patient experience of care as the ultimate strategy, and providing the appropriate resources to establish a highly reliable and safe environment. While previously boards have confined their role to quality oversight through dashboards and measurement, they must now extend this approach to include building the organizational culture with physicians and other clinicians that allows optimal clinical care to be delivered effectively. The board's relentless pursuit of quality will appeal to physicians' core professional values. Physicians who recognize this concern for quality in all the board's decisions and actions should develop more trust in the organization and become more willing collaborators.

Communication, as Alexander and Young indicate, is another critical lever to create collaboration. Yet it is not just clear and unfettered communication between the board and the medical staff that is necessary but also clear communication throughout the organization: clinician to clinician, clinician to staff, clinician to patient, and management to clinicians. The board must realize that physicians and other clinicians are often not trained in effective communication. By providing the resources to improve communications and teamwork, the board can demonstrate its commitment to working with physicians as partners in care delivery.

While the board cannot dictate the tenets of medical professionalism, it can establish the principles so that clinical practice in a complex medical delivery system requires both teamwork and effective communication. No single individual can reliably deliver the care necessary to achieve high quality outcomes. By practicing team leadership with management and the medical staff, the board members can model the team behaviors they expect of physicians who practice in their organization. This exhibition of governance professionalism is essential in gaining the medical staff's trust and confidence and recruiting them into the service of the organization's mission.

Leveraging what the authors call "workaround" organizational structures is another opportunity to increase physician alignment and collaboration, but there is a caveat here for governance. While these organizations may better align the physicians' and organization's incentives, the board must be careful that these arrangements are consistent with and further the hospital's mission. There must be a careful exploration of any unintended consequences such as isolation of the unaffiliated physicians, exclusion of the uninsured, and diminution of the necessary services that are poorly reimbursed. The board's fidelity to the hospital or health system's mission must not be compromised by ensuring alignment of financial incentives with physicians.

In the chapter's final section the authors offer four recommendations. Two of these can be viewed as change in the external environment that could facilitate physician engagement and partnership. Trustees, as advocates for their hospitals and communities, can work at a grassroots level to influence reimbursement policies and legal/regulatory requirements to provide common incentives and remove barriers to better physician and hospital integration. The other two recommendations are under more direct control of the governing body. Moving the medical staff organization from a representational forum to a body of collective accountability will require that the board set a priority for the organization to work collectively with its physicians in developing a new compact centered on the patient and built on mutual accountability. This activity will require board-dedicated time and resources. The board should take the lead in working with management and physicians to delineate expectations, responsibilities, and accountabilities. The result of this activity should be a new understanding that the organization and its physicians are accountable to the patients and communities they serve and that all their governance structures should be designed to achieve that goal.

One additional recommendation from Alexander and Young is for the board to develop its skills in strengthening the physician-hospital relationship. The American Hospital Association's Center for Healthcare Governance, through its Blue Ribbon Panel on Trustee Core Competencies, has recommended that all boards include individuals that have a working knowledge of: 1) health care and the delivery system; 2) business and finance; and 3) human resources and organizational development.[1] Each of these skill sets would allow board members to—in the authors' words—"reach out to medical staff members and cultivate a culture that embraces them." Boards need more than just the understanding of the clinical enterprise. They also need the expertise to help the organization

---

[1]Center for Healthcare Governance, *Competency-Based Governance: A Foundation for Board and Organizational Effectiveness*, The American Hospital Association, Chicago, IL, 2009, http://www.americangovernance.com/americangovernance/BRP/files/brp-2009.pdf

and its medical staff to develop a culture that can advance high-quality, safe, and reliable care while exercising sound business judgment to sustain the mission.

As hospitals and health systems evolve into more accountable care organizations, boards will need the skills to manage multiple relationships, not just with physicians but with other health care providers who support the continuum of care. The challenge will be similar to the one they currently face with physicians: to engage these new partners in efficient and effective care delivery while not losing sight of the core mission to improve the health of patients and communities.

CHAPTER EIGHT

OVERCOMING BARRIERS TO IMPROVED COLLABORATION AND ALIGNMENT

Cultural Issues

Katherine A. Schneider

[A] people is judged by history according to its contribution to the culture of other peoples flourishing at the same time and according to its contribution to the cultures which arise afterwards.

T. S. ELIOT, *NOTES TOWARDS THE DEFINITION OF CULTURE*

Introduction

Culture can be defined as learned, shared, patterns of behavior and beliefs. This chapter addresses the significant cultural differences between physicians and hospital leaders that will need to be overcome (or at least understood) to improve collaboration between the two entities. In order to achieve greater alignment and integration between physicians and hospitals, physicians must become and stay engaged, regardless of the financial and legal structure of the model. Engagement—a mutual commitment and degree of connectedness to a system—depends upon a level of shared vision, but even more so a high degree of trust. These factors may be seen as key differentiators in success-ful physician-hospital collaborations and in the related health outcomes for a community.

Building an environment of trust between hospitals and physicians requires recognition of and respect for cultural differences, identification of shared goals, and leveraging the strengths that each brings to the table to achieve those goals. Much has been written about the difficulties of bridging culture gaps between

The author gratefully acknowledges Bob Kiely, Jeff Brenner, MD, and Marilouise Venditti, MD, for their input.

physicians and administrators.[1] There have been numerous high-profile examples of conflicts of "white coats versus dark suits" that have led to major organizational disruptions.

The physician executive career path was initially driven by the need for a professional liaison role between medical staff and administration. The traditional job description for a vice president of medical affairs has all too often been summed up as "herding cats," a thankless activity that often results in isolation from both medical staff and hospital administration.[2] As these roles evolve to require both academic credentials (for example, an MBA degree) and clinical experience, physician leaders with significant operational authority and accountability may be better positioned to successfully lead the changes needed in the current reform environment.[3] In fact, ample evidence supports the positive organizational impact of strong clinical leadership, despite the general dearth of leadership development opportunities and incentives for physicians.[4] It is no coincidence that the health systems currently being looked to as best practice benchmarks of quality and efficiency (for example, Geisinger, Kaiser Permanente, Mayo, the Veterans Health Administration) all share the common characteristic of historical or current top-level physician leadership.

This chapter will first describe some of the main features of both hospital and physician culture, highlighting not only inter- and intragroup differences but also approaches to finding common ground. Rules *for* engagement will be proposed to assist in building empathy and trust (as opposed to battlefield rules *of* engagement). Next, a case study of Middlesex Hospital in Connecticut will illustrate how a hospital and a community of independent physicians have overcome cultural differences and successfully achieved alignment, with processes and results on a par with fully integrated delivery systems. The chapter concludes with a summary of lessons learned to help guide future efforts in physician-hospital integration, particularly in the common setting of a nonemployed medical staff.

Key Differences Between Hospital and Physician Cultures

The blue "H" highway sign, present in thousands of communities across the country, directs those in need to services, regardless of ability to pay, often with doors having been open continuously to serve the community for greater than a century. Community hospital archives abound with photographs and stories of founding physicians and philanthropists and quaint memorabilia, such as handwritten bills for a few dollars for two-week-long routine maternity stays or overnight checkups. However, the exponential growth in the past few decades of both the technological and administrative complexity of health care has driven major corporatization of the hospital industry.

Although economies of scale are predicted to lead to more mergers, acquisitions, and hospital megasystems, health care is fundamentally local due to its intimate nature—which several noted health care executives have often described as a "healing chain of trusting relationships."[5] The corporate culture that strives for performance excellence will neither achieve nor sustain it without nurturing loyalty from the local community or communities the organization serves.

Hospital leaders have to juggle simultaneous accountability to multiple stakeholders with competing agendas—boards, employees (possibly unions), community leaders, partners, multiple layers of regulators, physicians, patients, and payers. Top administrators are rewarded for leadership and strategic success, which produces desired outcomes in finance, customer and employee satisfaction, and quality. The focus on quality is largely around reducing variation in treatment patterns among patients (for example, use of clinical pathways to ensure adherence to checklists of evidence-based processes).[6]

Hospital administrators' work takes place through team meetings, committee meetings, board meetings, and more meetings. Although these are a mainstay of the workday for a hospital executive, for most physicians, every minute removed from direct patient care is money lost and time wasted (in other words, not their "real" work). A hospital executive's career path, by definition, is not characterized by a great deal of longevity—success leads to promotion upward or onward; failure leads to movement out. This is in contrast to a typical physician's career, particularly in specialties based on referrals or continuity of care, in which a successful practice builds equity by cultivating long-term relationships and local reputation over decades. In organizations with high rates of executive turnover, physician engagement may be impossible as physicians (as well as others in the organization) quickly learn that it is easier to wait out the tenure of an uncooperative or disliked hospital executive than to invest in collaboration.

Perhaps the biggest cultural challenge in achieving broad integration between hospitals and physicians is that the differences among physicians themselves are at least as great as those between any specific group of physicians and the hospital. In the best cases, these differences can guide development of a model that offers numerous options for physicians, rather than a one-size-fits-all dictum. In the worst cases, competing agendas and mistrust among physicians create a dysfunctional environment in which the integration conversation cannot even begin.

The degree of competition in a local market can also affect relationships among physicians, and between physicians and hospitals. Clearly, when a hospital and its affiliated physicians are the only game in town, the environment is more conducive to coordinated care than it is in a more competitive market. The physician culture differences between communities that can lead to radical variations in care have received a great deal of public attention only recently but such culture differences also play out within individual communities.[7]

The differences between primary care physicians and specialists (particularly hospital based) are the most recognized and play out in any multispecialty physician organization, including but not limited to traditional medical staffs. This has become particularly pronounced as primary care has, in many communities, moved completely out of the inpatient setting, and physician and hospital leaders struggle to redefine and maintain these relationships. For a completely office-based primary care physician, even the language of *physician-hospital integration* needs to be reframed as *system of care*, to deemphasize polarity and increase relevance to the daily workflow.

The differences between primary care physicians and many specialists relate not only to the daily skills and work setting but also to their perception of threat associated with a proposed hospital collaboration. The primary care physician's business—at least historically but perhaps less so recently—depends on continuity of the physician-patient relationship. Primary care physicians will thus react negatively to proposed hospital collaboration if they feel it devalues or diminishes that relationship by inserting institutional processes or systems. A proceduralist or acute care specialist relies on relationships with other physicians to control the flow of business, and the patient relationship may be comparatively shorter term (as treatment of an acutely ill patient requires daily, hourly, or nearly instantaneous decisions). Therefore loss of control within either of those workflows (referrals or clinical decision making) will create distress and distrust.

Generational differences are an emerging challenge in any workforce, and physicians are no exception.[8] The now mostly retired World War II generation was more comfortable with authority-based organizations than are the Baby Boomers, who are now at peak leadership age. In turn, the Baby Boomers question the work ethic of the Generation Xers, who seek a better life-work balance than their parents had and may be much more interested in employment than private practice. Layered onto this is the significant number of first-generation immigrants in the physician community, coming from a diverse array of backgrounds and experiences with other systems of health care, and in many cases having overcome challenges unthinkable to American-born colleagues. Although obviously generalizations, all of these differences must be accounted for in a physician engagement strategy—especially when physician leaders at the hospital table may not adequately reflect or represent the profile of the entire physician community.

Despite all of this, there is enough common ground underlying physician cultures to give hospital administrators guidance in building an environment of trust and respect. The years of demanding training, educational debt, and deferred gratification required to become a physician are arguably unparalleled and define physicians' self-image as professionals. However, physicians are essentially paid for technical piecework and rarely rewarded or recognized for professionalism (meticulous adherence to "doing the right thing," above and beyond "doing things right" technically).[9] This leads to cognitive dissonance, demoralization, and burnout for those trying to remain true to those values. Furthermore, years of school and training that traditionally value autonomy and reward task-based individual performance do not prepare physicians to function where reward is based on team or system success.[10] Similarly, physicians are trained to focus on patients as individuals, not populations, ideally practicing the combined science and art of medicine through their relationships with each unique patient. Organizational cultures that lean toward industrial models where physicians are "providers" and patients are commodities are anathema to most physicians.

Unfortunately, two effective organizational tools have not historically been included in physician education and are thus difficult to find in the physician culture and skill set. Virtually no physician practices, except those that are large or highly capitalized, engage in formal long-term strategic planning. Likewise, systematic quality improvement (as opposed to quality assurance) is unusual in typical small physician practices. Strategic planning and quality improvement are the building blocks of change, allowing an organization to ask, "Why should we change?" "How should we change?" and, "Is change working?" The usual view of physicians as risk averse and change resistant must be taken in this context—until now there has been little reason to change and few formal skills for managing change, let alone leading it.

In a review of a previous version of this chapter, a chief medical officer colleague warned of the offensive potential of the author's suggestion that instead of cat herding, a better animal metaphor for the work of physician leadership would be trying to get the attention of a hamster on a wheel, noting that "comparison to a cat suggests a cunning intelligence and independence—as opposed to a dumb rodent." However, a very progressive yet demoralized family physician colleague who recently left a model patient-centered medical home solo practice disagreed: "I have felt like a hamster on a wheel every day," he said. The ideal analogy for the challenge of engaging today's physicians in system change might be the task of asking a highly trained but exhausted athlete on a treadmill to change his or her workout gear in midrun, while simultaneously turning up the speed.

Though the hospital industry is hardly the gold standard for organizational agility and change management, the current imperative for change in the environment of health reform may represent the biggest win-win opportunity for physician engagement. Hospitals that can step up as trustworthy partners with organizational skills that can help support physician adaptation to a new environment will reap the benefits of alignment.

Simple Rules for Engagement

The clinician's training begins with a massive intake of factual science, then application of this knowledge in a highly structured, systematic, linear fashion. The presenting problem (chief complaint) is broken down through data collection into a set of possible next steps (differential diagnosis), which lead to explicit or implicit protocols learned through years of repetition—almost literally achievable in one's sleep. In contrast, the administrator's training consists of a combination of theoretical models and specific management skills (for example, finance, planning, marketing) that require deployment based on less clear-cut scientific evidence. The physician's role is generally geared toward fixing or preventing problems and avoiding harm. Operationally, the administrator's role includes putting out fires, but at a higher level it is about vision, opportunity, and breakthrough performance.

Despite these very different developmental histories, successful physicians and administrators can be viewed as sharing a common analytical skill set of understanding complex adaptive systems—the human organism and the large organization. Though they use different language and metrics, both are able to combine disciplined use of data (for example, vital signs and laboratory results or dollars and defect rates) with intuitive and qualitative skills (art of medicine or art of leadership). These skills are deployed to monitor the health of the patient or organization, diagnose problems early, effectively intervene, and demonstrate outcomes to stakeholders.

Complex adaptive systems can be guided fundamentally by a small number of simple rules. Achievement (or at least alignment) of a common mission, vision, and set of values can provide the simple rules to guide progress toward a less fragmented health care system. Trust is the essential element required to overcome differences, and transparency is key to establishing trust. When cynical assumptions are made in both camps regarding motives, progress is challenging, if not impossible. It is common for physicians to perceive hospital administrators as "green eyeshade" bureaucrats motivated solely by the bottom line, and for administrators, in turn, to perceive physicians as being motivated solely by their own financial interest. The actual motivations of both parties are likely to be more complicated, however. Explicit statements of motivating factors for and against engaging in collaboration and change should build trust through improved mutual understanding.

For the frontline physician, there are four simple rules for engagement with any external entity, at least one of which must be met in order to merit diversion of attention away from minute-to-minute patient care.

1. This must save me time.
2. This must add value to my patient's outcome.
3. This must noticeably increase my income or quality of life.
4. This must add to my professional satisfaction outside of the above.

Much of the time when administrators hope to involve physicians in initiatives of importance to hospitals, either none of the above apply or the case is not made compellingly. A family physician who no longer provides inpatient care is not going to show up for medical staff meetings that review new hospital policies, but she may be an enthusiastic participant in a forum on access to care or a faithful attendee at events that allow a rare opportunity to socialize with colleagues.

Physician participation in hospital-based quality measurement initiatives is an example of a situation in which the rules for engagement can be met. Physicians may debate the science and effect of specific measures and complain about burdensome new processes implemented without their input. However, the majority of physicians do not overtly resist being given convenient tools (rule no. 1) that are generally agreed to improve patient outcomes (rule no. 2), resulting in external recognition as being part of a high-quality system (rule no. 4), even without an immediate financial incentive.

On the flip side, for physicians frustrated by perceived lack of attention or inertia from hospital administration, a parallel set of rules can provide perspective. A physician may be a passionate advocate for adoption of a new process or technology to benefit his or her patients, and feel disenfranchised by administrators who do not act on this expert clinical advice. The administrator, on the other hand, is likely facing a slew of such requests and trying to balance politics, an uncooperative budget, and a shortage of staff—all prior to an impending unannounced site visit from a regulatory body. Accordingly, for engagement with physicians to be worth administrators' efforts, the activity must meet at least one of the following criteria:

1. This must be consistent with our organization's mission, vision, values, or strategy.
2. This must result in improvement in a key measurable outcome, particularly a publicly reported one, without adversely affecting another key measure.
3. This must result in increased happiness of a key stakeholder (for example, board member, patients, regulator, physician group, workforce, business partner) without resulting in ire from another one.
4. The operational requirements and implications must be adequately identified, and it must be possible to accommodate them.

The increasingly contentious issue of physicians requesting pay for emergency call is a perfect example of the lack of alignment that results when the rules for engagement are not met on both sides. From the administrator's perspective, having physicians voluntarily take emergency room call is critically important. Lack of access to appropriate emergency medical care creates immediate regulatory and legal risk. However, paying for emergency room call may not be economically feasible.

On the physician side, unless an independent physician is truly hungry for new business at any cost, emergency room call is likely to disrupt care of existing patients, take time away from family and sleep, increase legal exposure, and pay unreliably. Unlike the hospital, the physician does not enjoy the benefit of tax-exempt status in return for serving all who walk through the door.

Interestingly, the emergency room call dilemma crops up repeatedly in situations of dwindling hospital-physician alignment, resulting in a dramatic increase in the employment model (for example, hospitalists, nocturnists, surgicalists, laborists, and so on). Short of full-scale employment models, however, hospitals *can* successfully engage physicians in integration efforts as described in the following case study.

Case Study: Middlesex Hospital

The Middlesex Hospital experience and the evolution of the Center for Chronic Care Management are an example of where a shared vision of "doing the right thing" overcame cultural differences and persevered through market changes.[11] Middlesex Hospital is a century-old, community hospital in central Connecticut, with a typical mix of very small independent practices. Approximately one-third of the four hundred medical staff are employed. The employed physicians include hospital-based specialists (including hospitalists since 1999) and a medium-sized primary care group formed in the late 1990s by purchasing several small practices. A well-established family medicine residency program has supplied the community with a strong presence of family physicians, with approximately a third of its graduates practicing locally over the program's thirty-five year history. As the sole hospital in the county, with nearest competitors in urban settings a half-hour drive away, Middlesex has had a strong market share for core services, and a medical staff who by and large are not affiliated elsewhere. In addition to a 250-bed hospital, Middlesex also operates an ambulatory care campus a few miles away (surgery center, cancer center, diagnostics, and ancillary services), two 24/7 satellite emergency departments in the southern and eastern peripheries of the service area, a large home care agency, and an assisted living facility across the street from its main emergency room.

Around 1990, the hospital CEO position changed hands after physician-hospital relationships became strained past the breaking point. Bob Kiely, the incoming leader, describes arriving to find a core group of physician leaders who "got it," and who had achieved impressive outcomes, including a hospital length of stay consistently among the lowest in the state.[12] In the early 1990s, following Kiely's appointment, hospital and medical staff leadership came together with the independent practice association (with membership virtually identical to the medical staff) to develop a strategy and infrastructure to respond to increasing capitation in the marketplace. There was recognition that "we're stronger together," not only from a negotiation perspective but also because the clinical tools for successful financial outcomes *had* to be jointly developed and deployed across the continuum of care.

A joint physician-hospital entity was formed—Integrated Resources for the Middlesex Area (IRMA)—owned by the health system but governed by a board with physician majority. There was agreement in the principles of equity and simplicity—that tools and strategies should apply to all patients regardless of payer source, whenever possible. These tools included information technology systems, clinical pathways, and disease management programs—funded by the hospital and physicians through the revenues on joint commercial risk contracts begun in the mid-1990s.

Medical staff offices throughout the 600-square-mile service area were wired and trained to electronically access the hospital-based clinical data repository. This began as basic inpatient and outpatient lab and radiology results and grew incrementally to incorporate transcribed dictations, scanned emergency room notes, inpatient pharmacy records, EKGs, digital images, procedure records, remote electronic signatures, and eventually a full inpatient electronic medical record with physician order entry by the late 2000s. Though it initially met resistance, the information technology strategy was guided by a physician advisory group, which kept the focus on ease of use for the physician, reduction of duplicative testing, and access to the information most relevant to improving safe hand-offs in care.

A traditional utilization management approach, particularly for ambulatory care, proved to be a waste of resources and good will. Inpatient case management efforts continued to be so successful that payer denial rates were virtually zero, and eventually the top three commercial insurers granted the hospital exemption from concurrent utilization management review. (Notably, Medicare Advantage achieved almost zero market penetration in the area due to the original rate-setting methodology of using the already low local historical cost as baseline, making the region unattractive to health plan market entry.)

As capitation faded from this market, jointly developed clinical tools, such as disease management, were critical in supporting clinical integration. These efforts for commercially covered lives were strategically aligned with more broadly targeted efforts. In 2001 the hospital (as lead agency for a community coalition) secured a large federal grant to improve infrastructure for the uninsured. These funds were used to support disease management, low-cost access to pharmaceuticals, and a standardized system of assessing patients for financial assistance eligibility. Remarkably, this system was shared not only by the hospital and federally qualified health center but also by a large number of private practices.

In 2002 the decision was made to apply for the Medicare Physician Group Practice (PGP) Demonstration project, to further support clinical integration efforts and bring the fee-for-service Medicare population into alignment with commercial and uninsured strategies. Integrated Resources for the Middlesex Area (on behalf of the hospital and with individual opt-ins from 99 percent of the physicians) was the only network model among the ten physician groups selected for the PGP demonstration. The same year, IRMA was selected by its largest contracted commercial health plan as the only entity in the New England region to receive *two* Clinical Quality Partnership grants, in support of inpatient and outpatient quality improvement initiatives.

In the mid-2000s, joint payer contracting efforts ceased for a variety of reasons, including an increasing number of employed physicians and migration of a large primary care group to its own contracting platform. However, by then, much of the collaborative infrastructure was embedded in the system. The hospital and medical staff continued to participate in the PGP demonstration. Despite ongoing shared cynicism about the potential for financial reward from the project, physician and hospital leadership also placed shared value on staying at the leading edge of change and having input into their future destiny, particularly around public reporting of clinical quality.

Several other important delivery system improvement initiatives were possible because of the collaborative infrastructure that was in place. The primary care community engaged in two other competitive national demonstration projects, accelerating practice redesign. These included TransforMED and the academic sister project, Preparing Personal Physicians for Practice, commonly known as P4.[13] Competing surgical groups continue to be highly engaged in the American College of Surgeons National Surgical Quality Improvement Program (NSQIP) through partnership with the hospital. In the past five years, Middlesex Hospital hit the Solucient Top 100 list three times. *Dartmouth Atlas* data for care in the last two years of life for the chronically ill at Middlesex are in line with high-performing, fully integrated systems.

IRMA's disease management programs were the first provider-based programs to achieve National Committee for Quality Assurance (NCQA) accreditation in 2003 (in fact, the lead physician reviewer at the site visit pronounced his amazement to find upon arrival that he was walking into a hospital!). These community-oriented disease management programs in asthma, diabetes, heart failure, and smoking cessation differ in several key areas from the typical telephonic vendor-based program. First, they were developed by and for local physicians, as a three-way-care, face-to-face alliance among the patient, the care manager, and the physician. The programs were kicked off with physician and office staff education on evidence-based guidelines. Enrollment is through physician referral, as opposed to mailing and cold-calling based on mining administrative data. The care managers have relationships and inside-line status with the physicians and their office staff.

Second, the disease management programs were also developed by and for the local community. For example, a hospital board member—also on the board of education—served on the pediatric asthma program development committee. This ensured a linkage to every school nurse and school-based health center, and championing of the program's impressive results in reducing school absenteeism due to asthma, in addition to improvements in clinical and utilization measures. The program staff and leaders are also active in local and statewide public health and chronic disease coalitions, ensuring linkage to locally relevant resources (for example, the local Lion's Club funded Hemoglobin A1C testing for uninsured diabetics).

Developed initially to support joint contracting efforts, these programs were funded through those contracts and expanded through public and private grants into the Center for Chronic Care Management (CCCM), now one of the hospital's flagship community benefit and quality improvement programs. Furthermore, this infrastructure allows small physician practices to tap into care coordination resources required of a patient-centered medical home for those with chronic illness but otherwise out of reach for small practices. CCCM is open to all clinically appropriate patients of Middlesex-affiliated physicians, free of charge.

The Center for Chronic Care Management is an aligned solution to different challenges faced by physicians and the hospital. It meets all the simple rules for engagement for physicians by taking on time-consuming education and care coordination tasks, allowing physicians to perform physician-level work, and providing documentation and improved patient outcomes that are also aligned with several pay for performance programs. It meets the hospital's rule for engagement by supporting quality reporting, care transitions, credible community benefit, and patient and physician loyalty. However, although CCCM provides the ideal clinical infrastructure to support delivery reform, in the absence of a viable business model or reformed payment system, its sustainability is entirely dependent upon the hospital's financial health each budget cycle.

Conclusion

Middlesex's successes were built on a foundation of two decades of deliberate investment of time and money in building trusting relationships with physicians on a leadership level, through active listening, credible and open communication, and governance standards. Physician leaders are compensated for time spent away from patient care. These leaders are developed and chosen for their willingness and ability to make a positive contribution to the work—even if they vocally disagree at times, disruptive behavior is not rewarded. The medical executive and hospital board meetings are conducted jointly, and physicians and board members travel together to annual off-site educational programs to foster shared vision, mission, and values. As with any key infrastructure such as bricks and mortar or technology, hospitals that do not have the resources will be unable to make this investment in *social capital* as they struggle to keep basic clinical care afloat.[14]

As policymakers debate payment and delivery system reform, it is important to keep in mind the goal of greater integration across the continuum of care. Accordingly, differences in physician and hospital culture must be recognized and addressed. Key recommendations, first to payers and policymakers and then to hospitals seeking better alignment with physicians, are as follows:

1. Don't create polarization among physicians or between physicians and hospitals. (Unfortunately, this may be an inevitable by-product of episode-based payments and redistribution of payment in a budget-neutral fashion.)
2. Do create incentives for the specific clinical processes that are likely to benefit the patient first, even if these are unlikely to achieve immediate savings.
3. Don't allow competition and excess capacity in the system to increase fragmentation. The legal and regulatory environment (antitrust regulation, tax law, Stark laws, certificates of need, and so on) must be modified to allow collaboration that benefits patients and conserves resources (see Chapter Six).
4. Don't implement payment systems that reward relative performance rather than absolute performance (such as tiering rewards based upon percentile ranking). The latter will stifle sharing of best practices, information, and collaboration within communities with multiple providers. Quality improvement should be the tide that raises all boats, not a proprietary trade secret.
5. Prime the pump.[15] Getting the rank and file physicians to take time out of their transactional mode and redesign their work, even if there is significant future value, is extremely difficult without providing a noticeable up-front investment or other immediate incentive. This cannot be achieved through small, incremental pay for performance incentives unique to one payer, or per-member-per-month payments of a few dollars to support care coordination for a subpopulation of patients. Likewise, particularly for primary care and hospitals that are already struggling, health reform that changes

the rules of the game without investment in preparatory redesign will further separate the haves from the have-nots, worsening access to care, even without the added influx of newly insured patients.

6. Build trust early in professional development by integrating shared experiential learning into training programs for physicians and administrators. Residency programs are now required to incorporate systems-based practice into the curriculum, though many struggle to define this meaningfully. Administrative training programs virtually always require practicum work. Multidisciplinary learning opportunities for clinicians (physicians and nurses) have been promoted as essential for team-based care of the future, and this concept could and should be extended to executives-in-training as well.

7. Support a standardized, simple, sustainable system, yet one that does not dictate a one-size-fits-all model. Though hospitals are accustomed to administering a variety of conflicting payment systems simultaneously (for example, per diem versus case rate), physicians do not easily tolerate adapting their care practices based on payer or program of the month.

8. Make it clear that "the status quo is not on the table."[16] The provider community must understand that it has a choice of whether to be driving the train, on the train, or in front of the train. The delivery system has seen previous reform debates come and go, ultimately with payment cuts as the end game rather than substantive redesign. Fundamentally, physicians and hospitals are both on the delivery side of the equation, and their fates are intertwined. If and when they are credibly challenged with a new world order that rewards or requires alignment and shared goals, they will find ways to engage together to achieve shared success or else risk joint demise.

Much can be learned by further qualitative and quantitative study of existing formal and informal organizations. A recent conference attempted to dissect and understand ten communities identified as providing low-cost, high-quality care according to *Dartmouth Atlas* data. Common themes included a shared "moral compass" with focus on the community and a collaborative culture. (Other important elements included physicians well represented in hospital management, strong use of data, and a solid primary care infrastructure.)[17]

These common themes were not dependent upon a uniform structural model as an indicator of capacity for accountable care. Some of these attributes are clearly more actionable than others, and none is achievable overnight or without committed leadership and governance. Notably, however, none requires that physician culture be replaced or even subsumed by hospital culture or vice versa. Ultimately, alignment of a few key behaviors and beliefs can create fertile ground for successful delivery system redesign.

Notes

1. D. O'Hare and V. Kudrle, "Increasing Physician Engagement: Using Norms of Physician Culture to Improve Relations with Medical Staff," *Physician Executive* 33, no. 3 (2007): 38–45.

2. M. Glabman, "Physician Executives—the Lone Rangers of Administration?" *Physician Executive* 32, no. 3 (May–June 2006): 6–9.

3. L. Dister, "CMO or VPMA—Is There a Difference?" *Physician Executive* 35, no. 3 (2009): 12–16.

4. J. Mountford and C. Webb, "When Clinicians Lead," *McKinsey Quarterly, Health Care,* Feb. 2009, 1–8.

5. The author is grateful to her colleagues George Lynn, president-emeritus of AtlantiCare Health System, and Don Parker, president of AtlantiCare Health Services, for introducing her to this phrase.

6. Standardization of practice among physicians also plays out in cost-saving initiatives (for example, agreement on use of a single type of surgical device rather than having each physician use a different brand owing to individual preference and habit or training). Practice pattern variation among regions of the country has been extensively described by the *Dartmouth Atlas* project (see http://www.dartmouthatlas.org) and is widely believed to represent a significant cost-savings opportunity, as well as an opportunity for quality improvement. However, application of this information requires the ability to step out of not only the individual patient encounter point of view but also the deeply entrenched culture of local standards of care.

7. A. Gawande, "The Cost Conundrum: What a Texas Town Can Teach Us About Health Care," *New Yorker,* June 1, 2009, 36–44.

8. E. Berkovitz, "Understanding Your Changing Market" (workshop, American College of Physician Executives, AtlantiCare Regional Medical Center, Atlantic City, May 14, 2009).

9. Medical Professionalism Project, "Medical Professionalism in the New Millennium: A Physician's Charter," *The Lancet* 359, no. 9305 (February 9, 2002): 520–22.

10. R. L. Reece, "Twenty-Five Things I've Learned About the Physician Culture," Medinnovationblog, May 25, 2008, http://medinnovationblog.blogspot.com/2008/05/25-things-ive-learned-about-physician.html.

11. AHRQ Health Care, "Disease Management Programs Generate Improvements in Compliance, Adherence to Evidence-Based Processes, and Outcomes by Targeting Sickest Patients and Working Closely with Physicians," AHRQ Health Care Innovations Exchange, http://www.innovations.ahrq.gov/content.aspx?id=1903, July 8, 2008; R. A. Berenson, *Challenging the Status Quo in Chronic Disease Care: Seven Case Studies* (Oakland: California Healthcare Foundation, September 2006).

12. Personal communication with R. G. Kiely (telephone interview), Middlesex Health System, April 27, 2009.

13. TransforMED, home page, http://www.transformed.com.

14. Personal communication with R. G. Kiely.

15. P. H. Conway and C. Clancy, "Transformation of Health Care at the Front Line," *JAMA* 301, no. 7 (2009): 763–65.

16. B. H. Obama, opening remarks at the White House Summit on Health Reform, March 5, 2009, http://www.whitehouse.gov/the_press_office/Remarks-by-the-President-at-the -Opening-of-the-White-House-Forum-on-Health-Reform.

17. J. Iglehart, "Low-Cost, High-Quality Care in America," Health Affairs Blog, July 28, 2009, http://healthaffairs.org/blog/2009/07/28/low-cost-high-quality-care-in-america.

CHAPTER NINE

SPECIAL ISSUES FOR SAFETY NET HOSPITALS AND CLINICS

Benjamin K. Chu

Introduction

Safety net hospitals and clinics have a unique mission to provide care to all who need it, regardless of ability to pay. Financial support for hospital operations, physician and other professional services, equipment, treatments, and medications comes from disparate sources. The stability of funding depends on community commitment to the moral and ethical obligations to care for those in need. For the safety net, recruitment and retention of physicians in the face of such fiscal uncertainty is a huge problem. In addition, many communities served by safety net facilities are poor. High rates of poverty and population turnover in these communities present additional problems in recruiting physicians interested in caring for a stable panel of patients. The overlay of these special fiscal and socioeconomic burdens presents special issues for safety net institutions interested in building strong physician relationships. These burdens often require safety net hospitals and clinics to employ physician-hospital integration strategies different from those their non-safety net counterparts use. Successful models can offer insights into how and why hospitals serving a different population can approach tighter relationships with their physicians.

Public Safety Net Hospitals and Clinics—A Training Model of Care

Safety net hospitals and clinics, particularly public hospitals, trace their origin to almshouses. By necessity, institutions serving the poor needed to provide medical care to vulnerable populations whose economic circumstances predisposed them to ill health. The earliest models relied on physician volunteerism. A sense of civic duty and altruism was probably a strong underlying motivation.[1]

The variety of illnesses that could be found among the average poorhouse clientele naturally led to the use of these institutions as training grounds for new physicians. The evolution of the voluntary model of physician care to a training model served the purpose of educating the next wave of professionals while providing care to people who would otherwise have had difficulty receiving treatment. Senior physicians on medical school faculties and voluntary physicians who could get faculty appointments could benefit from having trainees support clinical care, thus freeing up time for academic pursuits, research endeavors, and expanding the clinical reach of the faculty member.

Public safety net hospitals that would otherwise have had difficulty recruiting and remunerating physician staff benefited from these arrangements. Young physicians who worked under the supervision of teaching faculty ensured professional services for the most vulnerable patients. These arrangements benefited safety net hospitals because, without a reliable payment source for physician services, the medical staff model prevalent in non-safety net hospitals was simply not feasible. Chronic understaffing, inadequate revenue and capital budgets, and the burdens of caring for the neediest also discouraged a private practice model of care.

In addition to the difficulties outlined in Chapter Ten with regard to physician-hospital relations in academic settings, public safety net hospitals that grew dependent on these teaching affiliations for physician staffing faced enormous difficulties achieving full alignment of physicians with the overall institutional mission. The teaching, research, and patient care focus in academia did not always align well with the primary mission of public hospitals to provide quality, patient-centered care. The primacy of teaching and research for most academic faculty combined with the transient nature of resident staff added to the difficulty for public safety net hospitals of achieving clear goals for efficiency, patient-centered access to care, and consistent, high-quality outcomes.

This early training model has been replicated in most urban safety net hospital settings. Public hospital-based ambulatory care facilities tied to safety net hospitals have also been the main source of ongoing care for many vulnerable populations across the United States. Community health centers, which also provide an important primary care base in many communities, rely on salaried physicians who have an acute sense of the social mission of these institutions or who have service obligations as a result of financial support during medical training. Community health centers that depend on physicians with short-term obligations for service run into many problems arising from relatively transient physician staffing.

Current Models of Physician Staffing in Public Hospitals and Health Systems

In 2006 the National Association of Public Hospitals and Health Systems (NAPH) published the results of a survey and a series of follow-up interviews with its membership. This survey, conducted for NAPH by the University HealthSystem Consortium, sheds light on current models of physician staffing for the public safety net and the strategies employed to align physicians to the larger mission of safety net institutions. The survey found that public hospitals employ three primary models to secure physician medical services (see Figure 9.1 and Table 9.1):

1. An *integrated model* of direct employment of medical staff physicians by the hospitals. In this model, physicians are integral parts of the operations, culture, and administration of the hospital. Theoretically, this model offers the greatest potential for physician alignment with organizational mission, values, and objectives. Adequate compensation, attention to performance, and aligned incentives with the public hospital mission are keys to the success of this model. There has been a recent move to modify the employment model with performance-based models of compensation to maximize incentives to achieve organizational goals. Most of these productivity-oriented payment reforms in the integrated model are not currently targeted to specific physicians but rather to a group or groups of physicians.

2. A *contracted service model* in which medical staff physicians are employed by a school of medicine, an independent physician group, or a faculty practice plan. The public hospital contracts with the medical school, academic medical center, or physician group for services at a rate that covers the physicians' salary expenses for clinical services. Performance and alignment of incentives to the safety net institution's mission and objectives can be difficult with contracted services. Incentive-based payment methodologies have been employed by many public hospitals. Most of these payments are tied to retrospective volume-based adjustments in payments to the contracted group, not to individual physicians. The potential to influence physicians to focus more on the key issues important to the public safety net institution is indirect. Another issue that hinders the effectiveness of this contracted service model is the exploding burden of uncompensated care that is the daily reality of safety net institutions. Even the most well-funded contract cannot keep up with the increasing demands for care without huge changes in the care delivery system and the system for financing care to the indigent and uninsured.

3. An *alliance model* of care that relies on physician billing for services to provide the financial backbone for physician compensation. Of course there are limits

to this mechanism to finance physician services, given the high burdens of uninsured and under-reimbursed services in public safety net settings. Many organizations employ the alliance model as a portion of the overall strategy for compensating physicians. For public safety net institutions, allowed fee-for-service billings for professional services might provide increased resources to support the mission. Risks inherent in this fee-for-service methodology could challenge the desire for better physician alignment to the public health mission of the public safety net institutions. However, if professional fee billing is used within a tighter context of the overall goals of the institution, the enhancement in revenues could be a major advantage. Productivity enhancements that are built into the incentive structure of the alliance model could also be important.

The following figure and table illustrate the potential of each model for greater physician-hospital integration in public safety net hospitals. As seen in Figure 9.1, the type of physician model a particular hospital uses depends on what the hospital seeks in its relationship to the physicians.[2] The two driving factors are the degree of integration and the ability to transform the practice or institution. Table 9.1 enumerates the positive and negative aspects of the three primary models hospitals have used to secure physician medical services.[3]

Regardless of the model used by the public safety net institution, the NAPH survey and interviews raised several issues. First, collecting and reporting data on the key elements of a physician group's business—clinical activity, service, and quality—is critical to running a productive and efficient practice. More

**FIGURE 9.1   CHARACTERISTICS OF MODELS
TO OBTAIN PHYSICIAN SERVICES**

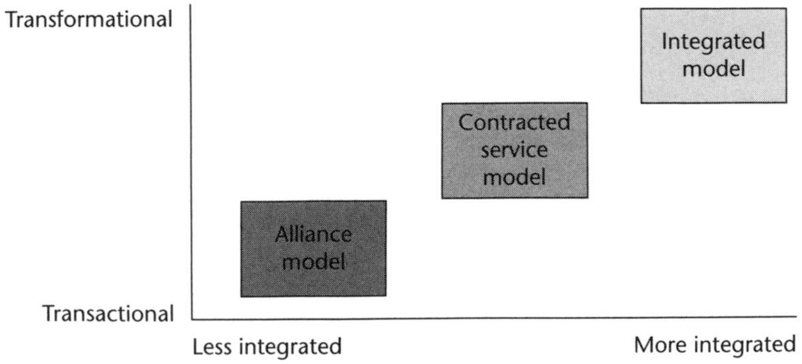

Source: University HealthSystem Consortium.

TABLE 9.1   THE PROS AND CONS OF
HOSPITAL-PHYSICIAN RELATIONSHIP MODELS

Model	Positive	Negative	Example
Integrated model	• Natural organizational alignment • Strong unified culture	• Financial consequences not felt by individual physician • Rigid to change • More difficult to track time and effort	• Denver Health • The MetroHealth System
Contracted service model	• Better ability to scale resources to demands • Easier to monitor and manage performance	• Lack of individual link to pay for performance • May not value other mission-related activities	• Parkland Health and Hospital System • San Francisco General Hospital
Alliance model	• Availability of clinical activity data • Better use of practice management tools • Flexible	• Lack of alignment between hospital and faculty practice plan physicians	• Hennepin County Medical Center • Truman Medical Centers

Source: University HealthSystem Consortium.

important than the collection and reporting of these data is their use in the management of the practices and the guidance they provide to drive for higher performance.

Second, careful accounting for and collection of physician-level time and effort data by mission (clinical service, teaching, research, and administration) is essential to understanding the true benefits of the academic relationships and serves as the cornerstone of an effective management program. Next, there is a greater need to develop systems to account for physician professional services. Most public hospitals lag in their ability to document and bill for professional services. This gap is a barrier to understanding what public safety net institutions are actually getting for the public expenditure for physician services.

Finally, the dependence on mission-driven and academic incentives for recruitment and retention of key physicians in public institutions masks the underlying difficulties in offering competitive compensation, especially for highly paid subspecialists. Recruitment efforts that capitalize on an individual physician's desire to serve a larger social mission have their limitations, especially when market forces are overwhelmingly pushing the doctor in a different direction.

There are inherent advantages and disadvantages to any model of physician staffing. Incentives are complex in each model. In public hospitals, the complexities are multiplied by the added layers of the academic mission to the patient care mission. In an ideal world, teaching, research, and patient care should come together to provide for the best services to the public safety net clientele.

Core Considerations for Physician-Hospital Integration in Public Safety Net Institutions

The public safety net suffers from the lack of clear outcome measures that have hampered the evaluation of the larger U.S. health care system. The recent drive to define and tie physician payment to clearer productivity and time and effort accountability measures only addresses a portion of the problem. Public safety net providers have a clear mission to improve the health of the vulnerable populations they serve, regardless of ability to pay. This mission is often tied to volume of services or availability of services without regard to the effectiveness of the effort. The ideal goal of physician-hospital integration is an aligned partnership that works toward greater effectiveness of care. The ultimate measure of success should not be volume or productivity based. Rather, the measures should be clear outcomes that have a reasonable chance of influencing the health of the population under the system's care.

The United States is a long way away from a system of payment that allows this alignment of incentives for physicians and the public safety-net institutions. As Shih and Guterman write in Chapter Four, the fee-for-service payment structure still rewards quantity of services, regardless of whether these units of service lead to a healthier population. Payment for an asthma patient is largely still tied to visits to the emergency department or hospitalization, rather than to doing what is necessary to keep the asthma under control to avoid unnecessary utilization. Productivity-based systems of payment for physician services must account for these misaligned incentives. When considering physician-hospital alignment in public safety net institutions, administrators must always keep in mind the larger purpose of these institutions is to act in the interest of the public's health, rather than the optimization of the revenue base of the institution.

Examples of Tighter Physician-Hospital Integration in Safety Net Institutions

Two safety net institutions are widely recognized as having successfully navigated many of the challenges related to physician-hospital integration. These are

Denver Health in Colorado and the New York City Health and Hospital System. Their experiences provide insight for other safety net institutions attempting to move toward tighter physician-hospital integration.

Denver Health

Denver Health was established in 1860 when Denver, Colorado, was a new mining town. In 1950 the city's Department of Health and Hospitals was created by a merger of the public health department, a visiting nurse service, and the hospital. In 1966 the Department of Health and Hospitals began implementing a primary care system, the Neighborhood Health Program, with financial support from the Office of Economic Opportunity, a federal program serving as part of President Johnson's War on Poverty. Eventually, the health system grew to its current configuration of eight community health centers and twelve school-based clinics located in Denver's medically under-served neighborhoods. These sites are fully integrated with other components of the Department of Health and Hospitals.

In 1997 Denver Health became an independent authority governed by a nine-member board appointed by the mayor and confirmed by the city council. A separate thirteen-member board governs the Neighborhood Health Program, fulfilling the federal grant requirement that this board be composed of 51 percent Denver Health patients. Effectively, the two boards work together to facilitate integration of the entire system. A Denver Health authority board member sits on the Neighborhood Health Program board. The chief executive officer of Denver Health regularly attends these board meetings as well. Although the existence of two boards might lead to conflict, there has been little conflict over the more than thirty years of the system, according to Denver Health's long-standing CEO.[4]

As with many urban safety net public institutions, Denver Health is a major affiliated teaching institution of a university—in this case, the University of Colorado School of Medicine. With a large complement of resident physicians, Denver Health nevertheless insisted on integrating its community health center physicians into the hospital and teaching operations. Over time, this full integration of the staff of the community clinics with the core staff of the hospital has enabled the system to achieve remarkable synergies.[5] It has developed managed care products that have allowed it to control the flow of dollars to the system and to drive care to more cost-effective ambulatory services rather than emergency care and hospital services. Recruitment and retention of physicians is markedly better than it is at the average public safety net institution.

Stable leadership and a stable physician base with aligned incentives for continuous quality improvement and improved patient outcomes define this system. Its recent dive into the use of the "lean" systems approach for improvement is yielding operational efficiency, the elimination of waste, and improvement in patient outcomes. It has invested in an information system that enhances the value of the integrated system, feeding critical information to teams who use the data to drive for better performance. The system has recently been recognized for its high-performance culture by the Commonwealth Fund Commission on a High Performance Health System.[6]

Denver Health is not without its challenges. This level of performance happens even while providing $318 million in uncompensated care in 2008. It provides care to approximately 25 percent of Denver residents, many of whom are indigent and uninsured. Despite this burden, the system is fiscally sound and a leader in the delivery of health care. Denver Health, as a safety net system, is far from a place of last resort but rather a place of first choice for many Denver residents.

New York City Health and Hospitals Corporation

The New York City Health and Hospitals Corporation (HHC) is the largest and oldest municipal hospital and health system in the United States. It serves 1.3 million New York City residents, including more than 400,000 uninsured people, through eleven municipal hospitals, four skilled nursing facilities, and an expansive ambulatory care network that includes hospital outpatient facilities, six large diagnostic and treatment facilities, and more than eighty community-based ambulatory care satellites.[7] It has a certified home health agency and a subsidiary managed care plan, the MetroPlus Health Plan, with 320,000 enrollees (as of early 2009). The system has provided care to waves of low-income New Yorkers from the time of the opening of the nation's first public hospital in the mid-1700s. This progenitor institution survives today as Bellevue Hospital.

The modern day HHC traces its origins to 1972, when the governance of the hospital and health system moved from the city's Department of Hospitals to a public benefit corporation whose members are appointed by the mayor. However, the corporation is allowed to operate with a relative degree of freedom from the politics of the city. Staffing for the municipal hospitals was haphazard and loosely based on a contracted model with the city's medical schools and academic health centers. These relationships were formalized in the 1960s under affiliation contracts, following a highly public review by the Piel Commission that raised serious issues with the existing arrangements.[8] In the ensuing decades, attempts to contractually obligate the affiliated institutions to provide greater accountability for the services rendered led to the development of greater reporting requirements and a faculty practice plan in six hospital settings that tied a significant portion of physician compensation to third-party billing for professional services.[9]

Finally a workload-based compensation model for the contracts was adopted in 1997. A crucial factor was the requirement in the early 1990s of a full-time medical director for each municipal hospital, whose job was to advocate on behalf of the HHC patient care agenda and to oversee the performance of the affiliate. These latest generation contracts also built in corporate-wide indicators covering quality of care, quality of service, quality of providers, and other metrics of performance. Financial repercussions for not meeting these metrics were also built into the contracts. This profound change in the affiliation contract to a workload-based model saved the system roughly 15 percent on a contract base of over $500 million a year.[10]

Not all academic institutions welcomed the changes in the affiliation contracts. Three hospitals that had affiliation agreements with academic institutions now contract with either a voluntary hospital or a professional corporation which employs the physicians. Many nonphysician services that had traditionally been contracted to affiliates were transferred back to HHC for direct management. Overall, these changes in the affiliation contracts not only saved precious dollars for the system but brought greater accountability for the quality and quantity of services provided. The changes not only resulted in higher levels of performance against objective measures but also improved productivity and morale in the hospitals as a result of providing a system of greater accountability, clarity of expectations, and improved service.

A by-product of the changes in the way HHC contracted for physician services in the late 1990s was the concurrent move to greater full-time attending presence in the hospital and clinic setting. Requirements for a full-time medical director and full-time chiefs of service were built into the early 1990s contract. The movement to a workload-based performance contract in 1997 accelerated the drive to a greater number of full-time physicians in the system. This included hospitalists in the inpatient setting, full-time intensivists in the intensive care units, and full-time attending physicians to provide care in the clinics, emergency room, and other areas of the hospital during the ensuing decade. Reasonable market-based compensation for physicians was also required for this transformation.

Recruiting and retaining physicians who are predisposed to the mission of the public safety net institutions was a crucial factor in the transformation of HHC into a high-performing health system. Clarifying the importance of the patient care mission relative to the teaching and research mission of the academic medical schools and medical centers was an essential ingredient. Another crucial ingredient was a two-decade investment in information technology, modern digital imaging equipment, and system-wide metrics of performance. The report on the HHC by the Commonwealth Fund Commission on a High Performance Health System highlighted the multidisciplinary teamwork that the system has applied to patient access, patient safety, and quality of care.[11] This continuous performance improvement culture would not have been possible without the changes in physician staffing brought about by the reforms outlined in this section.

A culture of change and high performance starts with a stable base of frontline staff and the clear priority of stable leadership to provide the tools to monitor, evaluate, and stimulate change intended to improve performance on behalf of patients. An additional benefit from the stability of physician staffing is the positive influence it has on training programs. The dependence of graduate medical education programs on volunteer and research-oriented academic faculty can lead to gaps not only in patient care but also in the teaching of residents in training. A full-time stable complement of clinical faculty leads to better oversight of residents and, ultimately, to better training.

What Can We Learn from Public Safety Net Hospitals and Clinics?

Public safety net institutions have always been a magnet for young physicians in training. Many are drawn to these institutions for the clinical experiences that come with taking care of some of the sickest and neediest populations. Others are drawn by the social mission to care for every person regardless of ability to pay. Physician recruitment for these institutions can depend on both the proximity of training programs and the altruistic tendencies of many physicians to help build medical staffs dedicated to the goals of public institutions. These natural advantages can, of course, be wasted without the clarity of purpose illustrated in both the Denver Health and New York City Health and Hospitals Corporation models. Several important lessons about creating a high-performance culture can be gleaned from these models.

1. Clear performance goals must always be articulated. Patient care expectations need to be at the forefront. Without these expectations, the teaching and research aspects of the academic health center mission will overshadow the public health mission of these institutions. Contrary to the greatest fears of academic health systems, accountability leads to greater rather than fewer opportunities for teaching and research.
2. Strong and stable leadership in the safety net health system is an essential component. This leadership includes crucial physician leadership that can carry forward the patient care agenda even as there is turnover in administration and hospital leadership.

3. Full-time physician commitment to the goals of the safety net is of paramount importance. Both Denver Health and HHC came to this important realization. An investment in full-time staff leads to better oversight of trainees and allows the institution to move forward with change efforts that can positively influence its culture. Without stability of frontline physician and leadership staff, a high-performance culture is difficult to achieve.

4. Compensation must be reasonably competitive to retain the best physicians and to achieve a commitment to performance excellence.

5. A commitment to delivery system innovation and change is an essential component of bringing physicians into a partnership for improved outcomes for safety net patients. Information technology and the willingness to push for delivery system changes to drive for better outcomes are key ingredients for high performance. A system focused on better outcomes will provide a more enticing environment for recruiting and retaining the best physicians.

6. Integration of primary care into the larger hospital and medical center is key. Without such integration it will be difficult to achieve the full potential of a systems approach to caring for the larger population. Both Denver Health and HHC have integrated these functions. The Boston public hospital system has also integrated the greater Boston area community health centers into its network. There are many other examples across the United States.

7. Physician-hospital integration is merely one step in a process to develop more vibrant care delivery structures to achieve better overall patient outcomes. The difficulties that community health centers have in recruiting and retaining dedicated physicians could be ameliorated with closer alliances with public safety net institutions and their academic affiliates. Governance issues can be solved, as in the example of Denver Health. Joint investments in information technology, care management protocols, chronic disease registries, and approaches to administrative oversight are all feasible with a greater system-level approach to the problem.

8. Cultural change will be the defining characteristic in any system of care. Physician-hospital integration is meaningless unless the partnership can be leveraged to achieve breakthrough performance in clinical outcomes for patients. This requires all parties to rethink the mission of the institution and their commitment to it.

Implications for Non-Safety Net Institutions

In thinking through the need for greater physician-hospital integration in the larger health care system, it is essential to keep in mind why tighter relationships are critical. At Denver Health and New York City Health and Hospitals

Corporation, the key driver was a desire to achieve higher levels of performance with respect to clinical outcomes and efficient care. Market dominance, fiscal stability, and other economic reasons may be the root of many efforts to integrate physicians and hospitals outside the safety net. However, economic reasons alone might not be adequate incentive to maintain integration efforts, particularly when inevitable choices must be made that require either the hospital or groups of physicians to compromise on financial interests. The failure of many physician hospital organizations (PHOs) whose basis for existence was purely financial points to the need for some higher-order objective for organizing.

Conclusion

Safety net hospitals and clinics may be able to overcome barriers to physician-hospital integration by tapping into their mission to care for all, regardless of ability to pay. In fact, the removal of individual financial incentives for physicians as a prime behavioral motivation might create more ideal conditions for integration.

With the prospect for significant health care reform in the United States during the next few years, the debate has shifted from a discussion of the potential for health insurance expansion to a realization that even with expansion, significant changes in the delivery system are necessary to produce better outcomes at a more affordable cost. Physician-hospital integration will be a key ingredient in this drive for greater effectiveness and efficiency. The public safety net hospital and clinic system has many significant advantages for accomplishing this integration. It also has the burden of responsibility for caring for the most needy and vulnerable populations. It has a rich tradition in academic teaching and research that cannot be a distraction from the larger patient care goals of the institutions. Success will depend on public safety net institutions putting in place the tools essential to drive high performance as well as making the necessary cultural change efforts to capitalize on these tools.

Notes

1. S. Opdycke, *No One Was Turned Away: The Role of the Public Hospitals in New York City Since 1900* (New York: Oxford University Press, 2000).
2. R. Brown, M. Keroack, and B. Tapper, *Strategies to Align the Performance of Medical Staff and Public Hospitals and Health Systems* (Washington, D.C.: National Association of Public Hospitals and Health Systems, 2006).
3. Brown and others, *Strategies to Align the Performance.*

4. P. A. Gabow, "Making a Public Hospital Work," *Health Affairs* 20, no. 4 (2001): 182–87.

5. P. Gabow, S. Elsert, and R. Wright, "Denver Health: A Model for the Integration of a Public Hospital and Community Health Centers," *Annals of Internal Medicine* 138, no. 2 (2003): 143–50.

6. R. Nuzum, D. McCarthy, A. Gauthier, and C. Beck, *Denver Health: A High-Performance Public Health Care System* (New York: The Commonwealth Fund, July 2007), http://www .commonwealthfund.org/Content/Publications/Fund-Reports/2007/Jul/Denver-Health-- A-High-Performance-Public-Health-Care-System.aspx.

7. J. I. Boufford, L. Gage, and K. W. Kiser, *New Approaches to Academic Health Center Affiliations: Public Hospitals and the Department of Veterans Affairs*, issue brief based on symposium sponsored by the Commonwealth Fund and the Robert F. Wagner Graduate School of Public Service (New York: New York University, April 1999).

8. G. Piel, *Community Health Services for New York City: Report and Staff Studies of the Commission on the Delivery of Personal Health Services* (New York: Praeger, 1969).

9. J. A. Barondess, "Municipal Hospitals in New York City: A Review of the Report of the Commission to Review the Health and Hospitals Corporation," *Bulletin of the New York Academy of Medicine* 70, no. 1 (1993): 8–25.

10. Boufford and others, "New Approaches."

11. D. McCarthy and K. Mueller, *The New York City Health and Hospitals Corporation: Transforming a Public Safety Net Delivery System to Achieve Higher Performance* (New York: The Commonwealth Fund, 2008).

CHAPTER TEN

SPECIAL ISSUES FOR ACADEMIC MEDICAL CENTERS

David Posch
Commentary by Darrell G. Kirch

Introduction

Hospitals associated with academic medical centers (AMCs) face unique issues in physician-hospital integration. Rather than having a singular focus (a patient care mission), AMC hospitals and physicians also have a research mission and a teaching or training mission, generally involving both residents and medical students. This tripartite mission of patient care, research, and teaching can be viewed as a strategic business advantage, in that on the one hand AMCs generally have the opportunity for multidisciplinary care coordination, early adoption of the latest technology or care innovation derived from research, and a lower-cost, high-quality workforce, namely those same residents. On the other hand AMCs' governance structures are more complex. There are also financial disadvantages. Costs related to postgraduate medical education are typically underreimbursed, and residents can add to costs because of clinical variability of practice. Further, AMCs often serve as community safety net organizations, with high burdens of uncompensated care.

Overcoming these complexities demands unique structures and systems to align the interests of all parties—the hospital, the medical school, and the faculty—in achieving superior clinical outcomes and academic stature in a financially responsible manner. This chapter examines the special challenges and opportunities facing physician-hospital integration in such academic settings and shows how integration has been accomplished in one AMC, Vanderbilt University Medical Center in Nashville, Tennessee. The chapter concludes with principles for physician-hospital collaboration, which might be successfully applied in other environments, outside of AMCs.

Organization and Management of AMCs

The basic organizational components of an AMC include hospitals, clinics, a school of medicine, and a faculty practice plan. The manner in which these components are organized varies greatly. Some AMCs have fully integrated structures with all elements part of a single legal entity, whereas others are made up of multiple legal entities. Depending on the legal structure, alignment of interests between the hospital, school of medicine, and individual faculty members (as hospital medical staff) can be challenging. For example, whereas the hospital may derive value from supply chain standardization of various high-cost implantable devices or appliances, academic research interests of the faculty may work against such standardization and favor technology innovation.

Mechanisms for intra-entity alignment are simpler in the fully integrated model, governed by a single board, with all members (faculty, staff, and health center administration, including the hospital) employed by the same organization. Alignment is far more difficult in a less integrated model where the hospital, school, and faculty practice plan all reside in different legal entities, with different boards and governance structures, and fully separate financial structures.

Hospitals are complex environments, demanding the coordination of the work of physicians, nurses, allied health professionals, and management. Every hospital, by regulation, has a *medical staff executive committee*, with numerous subcommittees of physicians, nurses, allied health representatives, and administrators. These may include subcommittees for credentialing, medical records, and quality, among others. Many hospitals also have employed medical directors, hired to ensure appropriate medical oversight of hospital functions, such as operating rooms, procedural labs, radiology, laboratory medicine, and emergency services. Finally, all hospitals have an administrative structure (generally a lay structure), normally charged with day-to-day responsibility for operations management, budgets, and plans. Thus, even small community hospitals have a fairly complex web of interlocking governance and management groups.

In addition to these complexities common in all hospitals, AMCs have the component of the university faculty hierarchy, with its deans, department heads, and so on. The faculty is normally organized into a faculty practice plan (or plans), which has its own governance and departmental management structures to provide the infrastructure to support the clinical care activities of the faculty. However, these departments also operate within a broader university context, with academic goals regarding teaching and research.

Although these multiple structures each serve a purpose in the management of the respective entities that compose an AMC, their multiplicity presents a challenge to efforts to achieve changes, including higher levels of performance. Coordinated, accountable leadership from both the medical staff (faculty) and hospital management must be present for the AMC to develop requisite clinical and business strategies, and to solve quality and cost structure problems. Residents in training must not only learn the science of their specialty, they must also see their teachers as role models of organizational leadership and cooperation for the good of the whole enterprise.

Financial Challenges for AMCs

In addition to having unique management challenges, AMCs also face special financial challenges. The leaders of many AMCs feel that they are inadequately reimbursed by the Medicare program for teaching activities. Such reimbursement includes payments for resident salaries and other *direct* costs (known as *direct medical education* [DME] costs) and payments for the indirect cost inflation effects of maintaining a training program (known as *indirect medical education* [IME] costs). A classic example is in the training of surgical residents in the operating room environment, one of the more costly environments of any hospital. Training during a surgical operation normally adds time to the case length, and extra operating room time is "money" to the hospital.

In addition, as mentioned earlier, the AMC hospital is often a key safety net provider in its community, providing care in an open emergency room and serving as a trauma center to all comers without regard for ability to pay. Such hospital capabilities provide important education venues for future doctors and other providers and help meet essential community needs. However, covering the cost of these services can be challenging. To be economically successful in such an environment, the AMC hospital must manage both case mix and unit costs, and do so with a quite diversified set of payers. Case mix is important to a hospital, because some services are higher margin generators than others. To achieve case mix objectives, the medical staff leadership needs to be actively engaged in managing the capacity of the medical staff at a subspecialty level, and the hospital administrators must supply the often specialized infrastructure for such high-margin services.

To achieve control of unit costs under most prepayment or episode-based payment systems, including Medicare DRGs, AMCs must tightly manage length of stay, labor, and supply costs. Length of stay is highly influenced by active, coordinated case management and adherence to protocols in writing and executing care orders. This task is harder in the AMC environment because of the cost inflation inherent in a teaching program. For example, residents order more tests than more experienced physicians.

There is also increased pressure in AMC hospitals to have a balanced portfolio of payers, with well-paying commercial contracts as an offset to underpayment from government sources. As the medical staff is the primary source of patients admitted to the hospital, such a diversified payer mix is dependent upon the faculty pursuing the same objective. Yet in this era of consumer-directed health care and direct contracting by employers, purchasers are seeking low-cost, high-quality options. AMC hospitals are often perceived by payers as being very high cost. It is a challenge to remain value competitive with non-AMC-based hospitals while still carrying out an academic mission.

These economic and competitive challenges create a real need for functional interdependency between the AMC hospital and its medical staff. The value imperative for the AMC is to find a specific competitive advantage in physician-hospital integration, especially by using this collaboration to make very visible improvement in quality and service, all in the context of a teaching and research environment.

Unique Role of the Medical School

Given the importance of faculty or medical staff behavior in achieving results in the AMC hospital, one other structural component bears closer examination—the medical school, with its academic departments, dean, and department chairs. In some AMCs, the medical staff may be organized into an independent practice group with departments organized for patient care purposes, and having separate academic department affiliations for teaching and research purposes. In more-integrated organizations, the medical staff are often organized into academic departments designed to serve all three missions (patient care, teaching, and research). In the latter case, the school, academic departments, dean, and department chairs play a dominant role in establishing the clinical goals and work priorities of the faculty. In the case of the former model, hospital management may establish goals for hospital performance in cost, service, and quality; but achieving those goals is dependent on medical staff performance as hospital *attendings* and in the supervision of residents. If the hospital's goals and those of the medical school dean and department chairs are not aligned, faculty behavior will be driven more by the imperatives of the medical school.

Medical schools, their deans and department chairs, and hospital departments in AMCs all have unique but overlapping interests. All have an interest in the proper education of students, residents, and fellows in various specialties and sub-specialties, not only for common mission motives but also because this enhances the entity's reputation. Similarly, all parties profit from research because robust research funding from third parties, successful bench and bedside studies, and frequent publication of findings also enhance the entity's reputation. An active clinical service supports both education and research ends because patient access systems and marketing are designed to match clinical problems to the unique academic interests of individual faculty members. Likewise, a sufficient patient base provides adequate teaching experiences for trainees and for the generation of research data and clinical trials.

Advantages and Challenges to Collaboration in AMCs

What are the incentives for faculty-based physicians, medical schools, and AMC hospitals to work together? Arguably, there is a financial symbiotic relationship between the hospital and the faculty in the academic enterprise, as the hospital is highly dependent upon aligned faculty and student behavior to achieve quality and margin results. In turn, the academic enterprise is dependent upon the hospital, not only as a training ground, but also as a funding source for the academic mission. Medical schools often rely on hospital financial support for the academic mission, as school-based professional billings, tuition, and grants usually come up short in providing funds for faculty salaries and other school costs and infrastructure.

In some systems, the school and faculty compete with the AMC hospital for lucrative ancillary income streams. However, developing a coordinated care delivery system with a shared funds flow creates greater value. The hospital or clinical enterprise is often the cash generator in AMCs, whereas the academic enterprise is typically a cash user. In nonprofit systems, excess cash from hospitals is used to meet community benefit requirements (provision of uncompensated or under-compensated indigent care), to recapitalize the hospital, and to capitalize the academic enterprise.

There are also important incentives for faculty physicians and AMC hospitals to work together around quality improvement. Performance improvement in the hospital, which is highly dependent upon medical staff behavior, leads to a better training environment and sometimes to better funding, as the institution's reputation for quality grows. As performance in the hospital improves, the entire AMC benefits.

The interests of the faculty physicians and the AMC hospital are also aligned around market competition with other hospitals. Schools of medicine provide an advantage through the research interests of faculty, leading to the early application of advanced technology and the development of unique health services for patients. Likewise, medical school affiliation attracts the best residents to the hospital.

Although synergies exist between the interests of AMC hospitals and medical school faculty, there are challenges as well. Successfully caring for patients with unusual or complex disease almost always involves more than one medical specialty. Strong department structures can be an impediment to creating the kind of multidisciplinary teams needed. Goals, time commitment, and incentives may vary from or compete with those that exist in the differing departments in which faculty members work. Such lack of coordination can lead to poor performance for the institution.

A management systems approach can assist in aligning the interest of the AMC hospital and its medical staff (or school-based faculty). The elements of such an approach include the following:

- Management and governance structures that pair physician and health system or hospital administrative leaders and create management teams for dialogue and problem solving
- Common or at least aligned goals among leaders in hospital administration and of the medical staff
- Metrics and transparency regarding operations, quality, and financial results relative to goals, with regular feedback
- Appropriate workplace infrastructure and tools to support the medical staff, residents, nurses, and allied health professionals in executing tasks associated with shared goals
- Alignment of physician-hospital financial incentives tied to goals with measured performance between administrative and medical staff leaders

To illustrate these points, Vanderbilt University Medical Center is used as a case example of the application of these management system approaches.

Case Study: Vanderbilt University Medical Center

Vanderbilt University Medical Center (VUMC), located in Nashville, Tennessee, is a fully integrated AMC. The medical center and all its components are wholly part of Vanderbilt University, legally and financially. Those components include hospitals, clinics, a school of medicine, and a school of nursing. The faculty medical staff are all employees of both the university and the medical center. In 2009 Vanderbilt University hospitals—inclusive of Vanderbilt University Hospital (VUH) for adult services, the Monroe Carroll Jr.-Vanderbilt Children's Hospital (MCJ-VCH), and the Psychiatric Hospital at Vanderbilt (PHV)—had 847 inpatient beds, with 51,831 admissions, and 102,998 emergency room visits (see Table 10.1). The Vanderbilt Clinics, both located on the same campus as the hospitals and medical school (and with sites throughout the region), had 1,250,000 provider-based visits in 2009. The clinics are the locations of the faculty's outpatient clinical practice and also serve as sites for outpatient clinical trials in a number of specialties.

The school of medicine has 392 medical students and 634 candidates in doctoral studies of various types. There are 636 residents and 223 clinical fellows. There are 1,908 full-time faculty members, 1,500 of whom are clinical faculty.

TABLE 10.1   OVERVIEW OF VUMC, 2009

Hospital beds	847
Admissions	51,831
Emergency room visits	102,998
Clinic visits	1,250,000
Medical students	392
Doctoral candidates	634
Residents	636
Fellows	223
School of medicine full-time faculty members	1,908 (including 1,500 clinical faculty)
School of nursing students	744
School of nursing full-time faculty members	214
Annual net revenue (FY08)	$2,205,144,000
School of medicine sponsored research revenue	$377,138,000
Value of uncompensated care provided	$245,300,000
Patient satisfaction: VUH overall quality of care	96th percentile
Patient satisfaction: MCJ-VCH overall quality of care	91st percentile
Patient satisfaction: willingness to recommend VUH	94th percentile
Patient satisfaction: willingness to recommend MCJ-VCH	91st percentile
Consumer preference for VUH and MCJ-VCH among local hospitals	No. 1

Source: Data from internal VUMC statistics.

The school of nursing has 744 students and a full-time faculty of 214. Collectively, the integrated medical center has $2,205,144,000 in annual net revenue (FY08). The school of medicine receives $377,138,000 in sponsored research revenue. The system provides $245,300,000 in uncompensated care. See Table 10.1 for a summary of these statistics.

Achievements

VUMC's hospitals have achieved superior results in a number of areas. In 2008 VUMC was named to the *U.S. News & World Report* honor roll of best hospitals, placing it among the top eighteen facilities in the country. In an article about VUMC, the authors stated that they "found a blend of pioneering and progressive skills, delivered with a healthy dose of humility and southern gentility and propelled by that all-too-elusive culture of excellence."[1]

In 2009 VUH was listed again on the *U.S. News & World Report* honor roll of hospitals, ranking at number 16.[2] Nine specialties were specially recognized: kidney (9), urology (10), cancer (13), diabetes and endocrine disorders (15), gynecology (16), otolaryngology (16), heart and heart surgery (17), respiratory disorders (18), and digestive disorders (32). MCJ-VCH had six specialties recognized among the top twenty-five of children's hospitals by the same publication in 2009: urology (6), neonatology (13), digestive disease (21), orthopedics (22), heart and heart surgery (23), and cancer (25).

In customer service and consumer preference, VUMC ranks high as well. Professional Research Consultants (PRC), a national health care market research organization, conducts proprietary satisfaction studies and benchmarks hospitals across 1,800 hospitals and health systems.[3] In 2009 VUH was in the 96th percentile for perception of overall quality of care, according to PRC, and in the 94th percentile for willingness to recommend to a friend. MCJ-VCH was in the 91st percentile on the same two dimensions. In consumer preference, measured in annual surveys by National Research Corporation (NRC),[4] both Vanderbilt's hospitals rank as the hospitals of choice against local competitors. Among local hospitals, VUH ranks number 1, with approximately a 30 percent preference score. MCJ-VCH also ranks number 1, with approximately a 50 percent preference score (see Table 10.1).

Financial performance of the medical center has also been solid. Earnings before interest, depreciation, and amortization and as a percentage of net revenue were 9.8 percent for fiscal year 2009. Volume has steadily increased, with the hospitals regulately operating at or near capacity. The clinics over the last ten years have increased their activity from approximately 575,000 provider-based visits to a forecast for fiscal year 2010 of 1,400,000 visits. Hospital admissions growth is now limited by hospital capacity, driving the addition of a new critical care tower of 114 new beds and twelve new operating rooms, scheduled to come on line in fiscal year 2010.

Finally, from an employee perspective, Vanderbilt University as a whole has achieved the distinction of being recognized as one of the top 100 employers in the country by *Fortune* magazine, the first AMC to have achieved this distinction.[5]

Results like these are achieved because of a number of factors. The performance cited would not have been possible without significant integration of the medical staff into the management and governance of the hospitals through paired management structures. In the model described more fully later in this chapter, specific aligned goals are established annually by and for administrative and medical leaders. Measurement is meticulous, detailed, regular, and transparent. Financial incentive systems are tied to these common goals. Workplace infrastructure, particularly the use of bioinformatics, assists faculty, house staff, nursing, and allied health professionals in executing evidence-based care plans.

Paired Management and Governance Structures

Administration of VUMC hospitals is based on a principle of paired leadership by physicians and administrators, with physicians holding the principle leadership position. A physician vice chancellor of health affairs/dean of the school of medicine leads the medical center as a whole (see the VUMC organizational chart, Figure 10.1). Associate deans and the various physician department chairs lead the medical school. The associate vice chancellor for health affairs/chief medical officer (CMO), a physician, leads the clinical enterprise. To this individual report the chief executive officers (CEOs) of VUH and MCJ-VCH (the CEO of MCJ-VCH is a physician), the CEO of the Vanderbilt clinics (who also serves as the executive director of the Vanderbilt Medical Group, the internal practice plan for the faculty), and the executive chief nursing officer for the system.

In the hospitals, physician chiefs of staff report to the hospital CEOs but also have a reporting relationship to the associate vice chancellor for health affairs/ CMO, with all working in a collegial manner. The Vanderbilt Medical Group has physician leadership through associate chief medical officers who work closely with the clinic CEO. This system of administration ensures the pairing of experienced administrative leaders with experienced clinical leaders in overseeing the direction and operation of the clinical enterprise.

The medical school department chairs are accountable to the vice chancellor of health affairs, dean, and associate deans, but also to the associate vice chancellor for health affairs/CMO, for their work that relates to the clinical enterprise. This paired management structure is mirrored at the level of specialty centers and departments within the AMC.

FIGURE 10.1 VUMC ABBREVIATED ORGANIZATION STRUCTURE

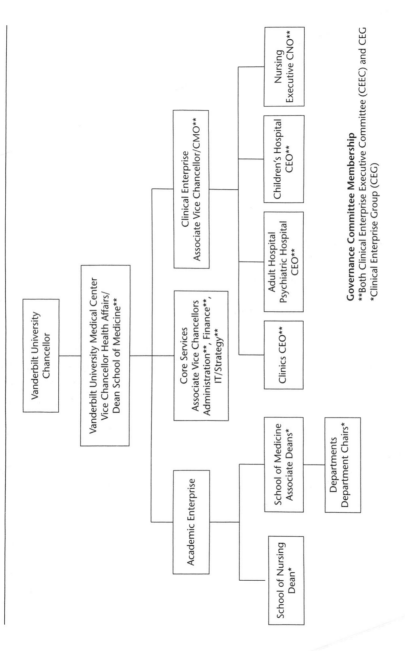

Vanderbilt University Chancellor

Vanderbilt University Medical Center Vice Chancellor Health Affairs/ Dean School of Medicine**

Academic Enterprise

Core Services Associate Vice Chancellors Administration**, Finance**, IT/Strategy**

Clinical Enterprise Associate Vice Chancellor/CMO**

School of Nursing Dean*

School of Medicine Associate Deans*

Departments Department Chairs*

Clinics CEO**

Adult Hospital Psychiatric Hospital CEO**

Children's Hospital CEO**

Nursing Executive CNO**

Governance Committee Membership
**Both Clinical Enterprise Executive Committee (CEEC) and CEG
*Clinical Enterprise Group (CEG)

Source: Author's analysis.

A number of governance structures exist to align behavior of these multiple entities, the first of which is the Clinical Enterprise Executive Committee (CEEC). The associate vice chancellor for health affairs/CMO chairs this committee, which meets weekly for several hours. Its members include the CEOs of the hospitals and clinics, the executive chief nursing officer, the chief financial officer, the system chief administrative officer, and various other senior leaders from the hospitals and clinic. The vice chancellor for health affairs / dean of the school of medicine attends as needed.

The CEEC sets direction and goals for the clinical enterprise, reviews performance, and initiates remedial plans as needed. This committee also establishes operating and capital budgets. The clinical centers and institutes report on a periodic basis to the CEEC, which functions as a governing board over these entities. The school-based department chairs that are related to a given clinical institute or center are invited to attend CEEC meetings when a related institute or center presents.

For example, leaders of the Heart Institute came to the CEEC to make the case for more clinical physician capacity, a realignment of the compensation structure, and the development of additional hospital capacity to include a hybrid catheterization laboratory and operating room. The leaders of the Heart Institute were joined at the CEEC presentation by the department chairs of medicine and surgery and the division chiefs of cardiology and cardiac surgery. The Heart Institute's proposals were attractive to the CEEC and required allocation of clinical enterprise capital and other resources. Also important, coordination was required between the clinical care activities and medical school departments, because department chairs must approve recruitment and appointment of new faculty. In addition, departments are responsible for physician compensation plans. The CEEC became the governance forum through which recruitment goals and changes to the compensation structure could be agreed on in the interest of the broader organization and hospital. The innovation of a hybrid cardiac catheterization laboratory (where interventional cardiologists and cardiac surgeons perform joint procedures) was made possible by the use of such a senior management oversight committee.

Whereas the CEEC serves as a forum for strategic decision making, another forum, the Clinical Enterprise Group (CEG)—involving more participants—allows broader discussions about clinical enterprise goals, performance, and alignment of interests with school-based departments of the medical staff. The CEG, which meets every other week, is likewise chaired by the associate vice chancellor for health affairs/CMO and is attended by the members of the CEEC and all the clinical department chairs, chiefs of staff, associate CMOs, and leaders of other corporate administrative offices (quality, marketing, and business development).

Major initiatives, goals, performance, and issues facing the entire medical center are discussed in the CEG, and work efforts are coordinated in support of those initiatives. In a quarterly meeting of the CEG known as Numbers Day (described in more detail later), the performance of the medical center and clinical enterprise is reviewed across several performance dimensions, allowing transparency of information among all leaders. Positive and negative trends are highlighted, opportunities for improvement are identified, and work efforts are coordinated. Follow-up discussions are scheduled to ensure progress toward desired ends and to identify and overcome impediments. Additional work is often delegated to various other medical staff committees subordinate to the CEG.

Aligned Goals for Administrative and Medical Leaders

The establishment of common measurable goals for administrative and medical leaders serves to align behavior. Vanderbilt, working with the Studer Group, adopted a scorecard methodology called a *balanced pillar approach*.[6] This approach organized goals around five pillars, or categories: people, service, quality, growth, and finance. (Recently, growth and finance have been combined and a new fifth pillar, innovation, has been added.) People goals involve internal staff and faculty satisfaction, retention, and turnover rates. Service goals involve patient or customer satisfaction on numerous dimensions with emphasis on perceptions of quality and willingness to recommend VUMC to friends and family. Quality goals focus on observed-to-expected mortality and other publicly reported clinical quality indicators. Another quality goal involves the elimination of medication errors and increasing the percentage of clinical orders being written in accordance with evidence-based order sets. Growth involves increasing the volume of admissions, office visits, operative procedures, and research funding. Discussions are held as to the size of various clinical services in relation to academic, financial, and market impact. Faculty recruitment objectives are then set based on these discussions. Finance goals include net revenue improvement, net income targets, and balance sheet objectives. Innovation, the newest pillar, involves specific initiatives to advance new care models at the AMC.

This aligned goal setting has achieved some clear improvements, for example, Vanderbilt University's making the Fortune 100 list as a best place to work—a multiyear effort. Another example is that VUMC moved into the top five AMCs for observed-to-expected mortality as measured by the University Healthsystem Consortium.[7]

The point of these explicit goals is to align behavior across the AMC. The medical and clinical executives and the clinical department chairs share many of the same goals that the medical center has as pillar goals. Each individual also has entity- or unit-specific goals for each pillar. As a result, hospital managers and medical staff receive consistent signals as to what needs to be accomplished.

Metrics, Transparency, and Feedback

Management committees and goal setting can be relatively meaningless without well-developed metrics to provide data-driven performance feedback to leaders. Discussions at groups such as the CEG are centered on dashboards and data reports of performance. As noted earlier, a quarterly Numbers Day meeting of all clinical and administrative leaders details the volume, financial, quality, and service performance of the entire VUMC. The consolidated results of VUMC and the results of every entity—the hospitals, clinics, schools, and school-based departments—are made available to all in Numbers Day books and presentations. Full transparency is the norm. Presentation of the data is followed by root cause analysis and discussion about how to achieve better performance.

Financial Incentives Tied to Goals

Shared and individual goals are tied to individual and work unit financial incentives. For over a decade, VUMC has tied a variable compensation or incentive program to the annual goal process for senior leaders, inclusive of all the members of the CEG. Variable compensation in the range of 20 to 30 percent of salary, depending upon position, can be earned or forgone based on measured performance against specific goals. Goals are established with threshold, target, and reach criteria, and the potential payout increases accordingly. Several years ago, this goal and incentive system was extended to include members of middle medical and administrative management with variable compensation at 10 percent. Finally, a success-sharing plan was implemented for the entire staff, providing a uniform bonus (to those not in the aforementioned plans) for overall successful performance of the medical center. The projected disbursement of these incentive compensation plans is included in the operating budget, and so an overall financial target is established which triggers the medical center's ability to pay any variable compensation. This organizational threshold has consistently been met.

Alignment of the interests of the medical staff—through the dean and clinical department chairs—is accomplished through the Numbers Day discussion. In addition, discussions focus on the five-year capital plan and the potential uses of funds for hospital investment and for academic investment in faculty development, research facilities, and related capabilities. Sources of funds for these investments are discussed, including debt and philanthropy. Also important, financial goals regarding results from operations from the hospitals and school are established. Because goals for the uses of funds are set to meet the desired objectives of the dean and clinical department chairs, these individuals are invested in the means by which these funds must be generated. Because hospital performance greatly affects medical school reputation and therefore revenue, medical school leadership support is aligned to the efforts required to generate budgeted hospital financial results.

Supportive Workplace Infrastructure and Tools

These systems of organizational structure, governance, goals, incentives, and data feedback align the interests of leaders and focus their attention in desired areas. But what of the work of the medical staff, residents, nurses, and other staff at the bedside, where millions of small everyday actions determine the quality outcomes for individual patients and the collective quality and financial outcomes of the medical center at large? Work tools and infrastructure designed to support the daily tasks of clinicians must also be aligned to AMC goals and receive the attention of leaders in capital allocation and in the investment of management time and effort.

Work at the bedside is guided by prior training, habit, a complex system of team relationships, and procedures often encoded in methods of documentation and computer systems. Although science and discovery advance, translating known best evidence into practice is a challenge in any environment. Excellent patient care demands a well-coordinated team under which the management of handoffs can determine the quality of care. For example, in most intensive care environments, numerous nurses, attending physicians from various disciplines, residents, respiratory therapists, and others interact. Substitutions of team members can occur throughout the day and during shift changes. The patient is under constant monitoring, as indicators of vital signs can change. Often information technology systems, intended to support care, are only used as basic transaction processing systems, which record and move data from one location to another. Instead, what is needed are decision support systems, which can guide behavior in real time. Such systems need to reflect known best evidence in practice to guide decision making at the point and moment of care. By use of such systems and through meticulous engineering of work processes, work habits can be changed and team coordination achieved.

VUMC devotes significant attention to work process reengineering and the creation of effective work support tools. For example, in the intensive care unit, a common problem for patients requiring ventilator assistance is ventilator-acquired pneumonia (VAP). Care for VAP-related complications is very expensive. The Institute for Healthcare Improvement has estimated the cost per VAP at

$40,000.[8] There are a number of known practices that can help prevent VAP, such as oral care, proper bed elevation, suctioning at proper intervals, and spontaneous breathing trials. The challenge in an intensive care environment is to not just spot check for such practices but to ensure continuous status and compliance. To achieve improved results, VUMC regularly hosts workshops of physicians, nurses, other health professionals, and information technology professionals to design new work practices and tools to improve care.[9] The result of such a workshop on ventilator-acquired pneumonia led directly to the creation of a real-time computer dashboard at the patient's bedside to inform clinical staff of patient status.[10] This allows the care team to have an easy visualization of results against a plan, which is derived from evidence. The outcomes of this effort led to a nearly 50 percent reduction in ventilator-acquired pneumonia and a 2009 number one ranking by the University Healthcare Consortium (UHC) in observed-to-expected length of stay, observed-to-expected cost, and observed-to-expected mortality for patients with more than ninety-six hours on a ventilator.

Conclusion

What are the implications of the Vanderbilt experience for other AMCs and other health systems with regard to physician-hospital integration? It seems that Vanderbilt's results are due to a special synergy of management and governance; aligned goals, metrics and transparency; financial incentives; and supportive workplace infrastructure and tools that do not exist at all AMCs, and that require physician-hospital integration at many levels within the AMC. Each AMC and hospital organization has its own culture and faces challenges because of its unique structural and legal arrangements. Incentives can vary greatly among the entities that make up such organizations, and the legal ability to align finances can be limiting (see Chapter Six). Each organization needs to analyze its incentive structure relative to the interests of the medical staff versus the interests of the hospital. Starting with the acknowledgment of shared interests, the first question to be asked is whether alignment of financial, quality, service, and other goals is possible at the AMC. If so, the next questions are these: Do governance forums exist to discuss and act to achieve such goals? Do internal politics allow leadership incentives to be aligned toward a common end? Are there metrics of performance and full transparency to guide performance? Can work reengineering be supported to change processes of care at the bedside? By using physician-hospital integration to successfully answer these questions, AMCs can improve their success in the future.

Notes

1. S. Baldauf and L. Lyon, "Vanderbilt's Special Mix of Skill, Passion, and Southern Comfort Hits All the Right Notes in Nashville," *U.S. News & World Report* 145, no. 2 (2008): 32–35.
2. Comarow, A. "America's Best Hospitals," *U.S. News & World Report* 146, no. 7 (2009): 84–112.
3. Professional Research Consultants, home page, http://www.prconline.com.
4. National Research Corporation (NRC) publishes the *NRC Healthcare Market Guide* and presents annual Consumer Choice Awards for the "most-preferred hospitals for quality and image in more than 300 U.S. markets"; http://hcmg.nationalresearch.com/Default. aspx?DN=7,1,Documents.
5. R. Levering and M. Moskowitz, "And the Winners Are," *Fortune* 159, no. 2 (2009): 67.
6. Q. Studer, *Hardwiring Excellence* (Gulf Breeze, Fla.: Fire Starter, 2003).
7. UHC Clinical Database, University Healthsystem Consortium, http://www.UHC.edu (accessed Oct. 13, 2009).
8. Institute for Healthcare Improvement, *Getting Started Kit: Prevent Ventilator-Associated Pneumonia: How-to Guide*, IHI 5 Million Lives Campaign, http://www.ihi.org/IHI/Topics/ CriticalCare/IntensiveCare/Changes/ImplementtheVentilatorBundle.htm.
9. W. W. Stead, N. Patel, and J. M. Starmer, "Closing the Loop in Practice to Assure the Desired Performance," *Transactions of the American Clinical and Climatological Association* 119 (2008): 185–95; W. W. Stead and J. M. Starmer, "Practical Frontline Challenges to Moving Beyond the Expert-based Practice," in *Evidence-Based Medicine and the Changing Nature of Health Care*, ed. M. B. McClellan, J. M. McGinnis, E. G. Nabel, and L. M. Olsen, 94–105 (Washington, D.C.: National Academies Press, 2008).
10. J. M. Starmer and D. Giuse, "A Real-Time Ventilator Management Dashboard: Toward Hardwiring Compliance with Evidence-Based Guidelines," *AMIA Annual Symposium Proceedings*, 2008: 702–06.

Commentary

Darrell G. Kirch, President and CEO of the Association of American Medical Colleges

The preceding chapter by David Posch clearly shows the unique space academic medical centers (AMCs) occupy in the nation's health care system, particularly when it comes to driving innovation. Today, as our nation moves closer to health care reform, AMCs have an unprecedented opportunity to lead the nation in transformational change. As Posch and other authors in this book note, improved integration among providers is key to achieving meaningful reform of our health care system. However, achieving the level of integration necessary to create greater value in health care delivery will require changing the current financing and delivery systems in tandem. With so many promising models under discussion—including the concept of accountable care organizations discussed throughout this book—and given the scale of disruptive innovation contemplated by their implementation, what is the best way to test proposed changes?

Working with leaders at its member institutions, the Association of American Medical Colleges (AAMC) has developed the concept of regional alliances called *health care innovation zones* (HIZs). In a HIZ, academic medical centers—with their aligned hospitals and physicians—would sit at the nexus of an integrated delivery network that provides the full spectrum of inpatient and outpatient care. Partnering with government and other stakeholders, and—as described later—freed of current reimbursement disincentives and regulatory constraints, these regional alliances would explore and test new business models of delivery and other innovations. The knowledge gleaned from implementing and testing HIZs on a regional basis would ultimately be used to more broadly improve the resource utilization of the U.S. health care system.

An important goal of HIZs is to demonstrate that coordination of care, coupled with a reimbursement model free of the counterproductive incentives and fragmentation caused by fee-for-service payment, supports more effective planning and delivery of services. Additionally, HIZs would allocate resources where they add the greatest value, for example, toward care for chronic and debilitating diseases. By using capitated or partially capitated payment methods to encourage collaboration, quality, safety, and cost efficiency, providers would see more effective utilization of their professional expertise; patients would receive coordinated, quality care; and a better balance in how and when services are provided (and by whom) would be achieved.

The strength of a HIZ would lie in its parallel implementation of new care delivery models and new reimbursement approaches. The ideal environment for a HIZ would include a variety of public and private participants, a large and diverse patient population, and providers with experience in managing capitated health care services. Each HIZ would be created by taking existing health care spending by one or more payers for large populations in defined geographical regions and using those funds to create systems that better align health care delivery and financing.

This type of realignment of incentives can be demonstrated only if sufficient flexibility is granted to innovators. To facilitate successful systems redesign within a HIZ, exemptions and waivers from certain laws, rules, and regulations would be required, including certain antitrust laws and other constraints that currently limit provider cooperation (for example, Medicaid and Medicare rules and regulations and other relevant state and local restrictions, such as scope of practice restraints).

Academic medical centers—through their tripartite mission of patient care, medical education, and research—are uniquely positioned to lead health care innovation zones. Because AMCs include teaching hospitals and health systems, health researchers, medical schools, and large, multispecialty practice plans, they can simultaneously play a number of roles. These include serving as conveners for achieving care coordination across the community, using educational resources to improve the balance of primary and specialty care, and leveraging research resources to measure and monitor the impact of innovations.

With regard to patient care, AMCs possess a breadth and depth of clinical expertise and have a long-standing track record of caring for all population segments. They also have an organized physician group practice of the size and sophistication needed to coordinate the delivery of the full continuum of care to a defined population. In contrast to the widespread fragmentation of providers, AMCs are large enough to provide the financial stability needed for system redesign and experimentation. Of great importance is the fact that AMCs lead the health care community in the adoption of critically important information technology tools.

As medical educators, AMCs train the next generation of health professionals for patient-centered care delivery and for work environments that are increasingly interprofessional. They also play significant roles in delivering continuing medical education to their community's practicing physicians.

The clinical and health services research capacity of AMCs would facilitate the collection and analysis of the valuable data that would be produced in a health care innovation zone. As new delivery models were tested, AMCs would be able to examine and share data related to quality and cost. Finally, each AMC would bring to HIZ leadership its long-standing history of community and regional partnerships, and a credibility that is unmatched by other institutions.

By testing a new business model that rewards outcomes rather than units of service, HIZs would help move U.S. health care delivery toward a system that rewards the maintenance of population health. Further, HIZs would generate greater value by delivering care in lower-cost settings, making providers, insurers, and patients partners in the use of resources and eliminating unnecessary administrative tasks that detract from the care process. In addition to improved integration, HIZs would provide platforms for faster access to health and billing records, aligned provider incentives that reward outcomes and quality, and consumer incentives that reward creation of new applications such as personal health records.

By bridging the *knowledge gap* that currently exists between conceptualizing and implementing a well-functioning health care delivery system, health care innovation zones would serve as the infrastructure for the type of testing that would enable true health care reform to be achieved. Regardless of what takes place on the political and legislative fronts, the AAMC and the academic medical centers it represents stand ready to move this innovation forward.

CHAPTER ELEVEN

WHAT NEEDS TO HAPPEN NEXT?

Francis J. Crosson

If the vision of The Commonwealth Fund Commission on a High Performance Health System is to be achieved,[1] this nation must change both the structure and payment system of health care delivery. Deeply embedded in this work is the task of substantially changing how physicians and hospitals engage with each other. The question is not, How should physicians and hospitals *relate* to each other? Rather, the question is, How should physicians and hospitals *integrate* with each other to produce the quality and affordability of care that the nation deserves? The work that must be done is not just about behaving better; it is about working in different structures, with different incentives, and with a different level of accountability for results.

In the preceding chapters, some of the nation's most forward-looking health care leaders and thinkers have described each of the many aspects of the current physician-hospital environment. They have detailed ideas for constructive changes—structural, financial, cultural, operational, and legal and regulatory—and provided examples of how such changes can be and have been accomplished. But one cannot imagine such significant change occurring in nearly one-sixth of the U.S. economy without the engagement and commitment of all involved stakeholders. This final chapter describes who those stakeholders are and, drawing on the ideas presented in the earlier chapters of this book, identifies specific actions that each group of stakeholders should undertake to set the nation on a path toward better care through improved physician-hospital integration. (These next steps are summarized in Table 11.1.)

TABLE 11.1   SUMMARY OF RECOMMENDED NEXT STEPS

Stakeholders	Next Steps
Physicians	• Create or join a multispecialty group practice • Adapt to new payment methodologies • Newly engage with hospital governance and management • Understand the utility of care and patient safety pathways • Manage the new reality of transparency • Learn to lead and follow
Existing multispecialty group practices	• Clarify what works
Hospitals	• View physicians as partners, not competitors or employees • Support the development and success of legitimate physician leaders • Build a business case for success with new payment models • Support the formation of multispecialty group practice
Payers	• Support payment reforms that move away from fee-for-service • Experiment with risk sharing rather than risk transfer • Accept reasonable delivery system consolidation
Government as lawmaker and regulator	• Mitigate legal and regulatory obstacles to integration • Prevent delivery system monopolistic pricing
Patients, patient advocates, and the media	• Understand the value of care coordination; expect seamless care

Source: Authors' analysis.

Physicians

Create or Join a Multispecialty Group Practice

Assuming that physician-hospital integration will be an important element of a twenty-first-century American health care system, physicians need to organize themselves rather differently than they have in many parts of the country. They must be partners with their hospitals, rather than antagonists or employees who feel disconnected from critical management decisions. Physicians need to speak with one voice across specialties, on business as well as clinical issues, or risk being split into ineffectual self-interested factions. In Chapters Five and Eight, Genovese and Schneider provide useful windows into the thinking of hospital staff physicians on this point.

There is no single successful model for this type of physician unity. There are a few very large multispecialty group practices (MSGPs), with over 2,000 physicians each. There are many more MSGPs that are smaller. Although there is no recognized minimum size, some observers believe that, given existing specialty-to-population ratios, about fifty physicians is a reasonable operating threshold, especially for a group seeking to form an integrated relationship with a hospital. Group practices can be housed in a common office space or distributed in smaller offices linked by information technology. Group practice physicians can be self-employed as co-owners of a group, employed by a group, employed by another entity such as a hospital, or semi-independent and linked by an exclusive contractual arrangement with a core group practice. There must be enough financial and cultural cohesiveness among the physicians, however, to support common governance and collective accountability. Not all physician-based contracting entities, such as many independent practice associations (IPAs), have these characteristics.

A shift toward multispecialty group practice will seem natural for some physicians and anathema to others. To many physicians, especially older ones, solo, small-group, or single-specialty practice is synonymous with complete clinical independence and a necessity for appropriate patient care. Others see group practice, especially salaried group practice, as less financially advantageous than a smaller practice setting. Still others are simply not joiners by nature, preferring to manage even the smallest details of their practice environment free from external constraints.

There is room for optimism, however. As some of the larger multispecialty group practices, such as Permanente, Mayo, Geisinger, and other have expanded in recent years, two trends have become evident. First, these groups are no longer attracting only special group-minded physicians. Rather, group practice seems more and more to be attracting a broader sample of physicians, including some in established small practices who ten years ago would never have considered joining a larger practice. This trend has been starkly evident in the San Francisco Bay Area, where significant numbers of physicians from local university training programs have lined up to join Kaiser Permanente in recent years. Some of this change appears to be due to an increasingly hostile payment and regulatory environment. But the second, perhaps more significant, trend is that the demographic mix of newly minted physicians has changed appreciably in the last two decades. Many more new physicians than previously are women, who seek group practice settings more frequently than earlier generations of (mostly) male physicians, as group practice lends itself more easily to a balance of work and family life. In addition, both male and female physicians of Generations X and Y appear to bring to career planning a different assessment of the value of independent practice than their physician fathers (and in a few cases, mothers) did.

Adapt to New Payment Methodologies

The rhythm of most physician practice has been driven for the last half century by the drumbeat of fee-for-service (FFS) payment. Practices survive or not by the volume of services provided. Among cynical physicians, the hunter-gatherer aphorism for this dynamic is "you eat what you can kill." As noted by Guterman and Shih in Chapter Four, this mode of payment is credited as a major force in health care cost inflation.

Prospective payment of groups and payment of physicians by salary have been less common. Nevertheless, there are enough examples of organizational success with both of these alternative payment models (see Chapter Three) to demonstrate their viability. However, for more physicians to be comfortable moving from FFS payment to something new, both positive and negative incentives will likely be required. As described in Chapter Four, public and private payers are interested in testing new physician payment methods and incentives, such as prospective medical home payments and bundled payments to physicians and hospitals. Further, if the development of accountable care organizations (ACOs)—as described by Shortell and colleagues in Chapter Three—continues, it should create opportunities for constructive shared savings opportunities for physicians in such entities.

At the same time, Medicare payments to physicians per unit of service have been nearly flat for seven years, and are likely to remain so.[2] In addition, indications from a number of health care reform proposals suggest that FFS payment rates for newly insured individuals from private and potential new public payers may fall below the expectations of physician payment advocates.

Forward-looking physicians and physician groups would be wise to begin to prepare for new ways of being paid for their services. There is evidence that some physicians are already doing so.[3] Physicians and physician groups so prepared and experienced will be more able, in turn, to participate as equals in physician hospital organizations seeking to thrive in the new payment environment.

Newly Engage with Hospital Governance and Management

As noted by Alexander and Young in Chapter Seven, physician-hospital integration will require a new hospital governance model. In California, this process has, perhaps, begun with the promulgation of Section 2282 of the *California Business and Professions Code* on January 1, 2005. This regulation, which followed an acrimonious dispute between a Southern California hospital and its professional medical staff, specifies that a hospital board may exercise its authority "in matters pertaining to the quality of patient care" only if it reasonably finds that the medical staff has failed to fulfill one or more of its patient care related duties. This test of *reasonableness* is new and represents a check on the previously held full authority of the hospital board. It has served to create a new level of dialogue between medical staff physicians and hospital administrators in some California hospitals.

Even in the absence of such regulatory change, it would serve medical staff leaders well to put aside the legacy of distrust and alienation that has characterized the relationships between these two different sorts of people (see Chapters Five and Eight), and seek to form alliances and develop common goals. Trust, which grows as a consequence of openness and successful cooperation, can provide the basis for negotiation of a shared governance role for the professional medical staff. As Schneider states in Chapter Eight, "Trust is the essential element required to overcome differences, and transparency is the key to establishing trust."

Understand the Utility of Care and Patient Safety Pathways

If the work of Dr. Don Berwick, Dr. Brent James, and others has shown anything, it is that the application of systematic care pathways in hospitals saves lives and money.[4] More recently, Haynes and colleagues—including well-known quality improvement advocate, Dr. Atul Gawande—have called for the use of operating room checklists similar to those routinely used in airliner cockpits, to reduce mistakes and resultant injuries to patients.[5] Such activities are seen by some physicians as cookbook medicine and a violation of physician autonomy to make decisions in the best interests of the patient. However, these attitudes have failed the test of field experience in recent years and no longer have a place in a modern hospital. The key to acceptance by medical staff physicians of safer and more consistent processes of care lies in medical staff involvement in the development and promulgation of these processes. This cannot be done if physicians are unwilling to participate with hospital nurses and nonprofessional staff in this work. As noted by Genovese in Chapter Five, "patient safety improvement initiatives . . . would be more effective and broader reaching if a greater level of integration between physicians and hospitals existed. The resulting joint goals, appropriate incentives, and breakdown in organizational barriers could produce results in patient safety with remarkable speed and efficiency."

Manage the New Reality of Transparency

Medical practice is moving into a fishbowl environment, and few physicians, or hospitals, for that matter, find it comfortable to think of being there. Historically, most medical practice was fundamentally self-policing, depending on professional integrity and Hippocratic ethics for the establishment of trust with patients. That is changing. New medical technology has empowered physicians to do miracles for patients that were inconceivable even for their parents' generation. But paradoxically, such miracle technologies can serve to distance physicians from those they care for. It can be as simple as the difference between a physician's thoughtful listening to a patient's heart and an impersonal referral for echocardiography. With this type of distance has come mistrust.

At the same time, the rising cost of health care services has pushed employers and health plans, as well as consumers, to ask for more detail about the care they are paying for. As a consequence, new reporting requirements seem to arise each year for physicians and hospitals. One of the ironies of the coming transition to electronic medical records is that it will make reporting of care processes and outcomes much simpler and less expensive but will also allow payers and others to examine a level of clinical detail that has never been available before. "All the better for improving quality," many will say, and be right. "Oh my, how intrusive!" many physicians will say, and be angry. But that is where we must go. Many physician leaders believe, correctly, that the best place to influence this movement is from the front. Group practices, both established and nascent, need to be present, counted, and counted on in the development of reporting requirements.

Learn to Lead and Follow

Physicians can be quite independent folk, often by both inclination and training. However, physician organizations, by definition, require leaders, and leaders require willing followers to be successful. Physician-hospital integration will require that physicians select physician leaders and then follow them. Hospital administrators deserve able physician partners if cooperative management is to succeed. Good physician leaders require training in business skills and time to exercise those skills. This may require financial support from the members of the medical staff, especially if the physician leader is to be seen as independent enough of hospital leadership. Similarly, medical staff physicians must be willing to give physician leaders a presumption of competence and good faith in decision making, unless there is good reason to withhold such support.

Existing Multispecialty Group Practices

Clarify What Works

Much has been made in the last few years about the relative success of multispecialty group practices (MSGPs) and integrated delivery systems (IDSs) in achieving high levels of performance on quality measures.[6] This book itself holds out the promise that such gains can be extended by such organizations and by newly formed groups, which is why physician-hospital integration is so important. Most payment reform innovations, as described in Chapter Four, are predicated on the idea that such organizations, whether ACOs or not, are likely to be able to achieve lower cost and better value for patients and payers if appropriate payment incentives are created for them.

What is less clear is exactly what structural and process elements are essential for this special flame of commitment to excellence to exist in these organizations. Physician leaders of multispecialty group practices and integrated delivery systems often point to such elements as multispecialty financial integration, physician self-governance, physician payment by salary, the use of an electronic medical record (EMR), the use of guidelines and hospital care pathways, formal and informal peer review, physician management and leadership capabilities, and cultural cohesion, common history, and common mission as critical to success. Most of these elements can be found to some degree in successful, large, integrated delivery systems, but Casalino and colleagues have found that even among IDSs, some such elements vary from site to site a good deal.[7]

There are essentially two paths to delivery system reform, (as depicted in Figure 11.1). The first path—Track A—involves fairly rapid development of new payment methods for established multispecialty group practices and integrated delivery systems. The idea would be to test quickly what the best existing organizations could do with better payment incentives, and use that experience to create incentives for more such organizations to form.

FIGURE 11.1   TWO PATHS TO DELIVERY SYSTEM REFORM

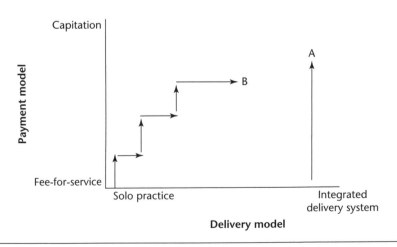

Track B involves a much broader but slower approach to delivery system reform. In that model, there is a more ubiquitous but stepwise approach to change, bringing many more delivery systems and nonsystems into an iterative process of incremental payment reform, then incremental structural reform, then more payment reform, and so on. Each track has its adherents. It is possible—quite likely, in fact—that some payers will be interested in seeing progress proceed down both tracks simultaneously.

For either track to be successful, it will be necessary to know more about which of the elements described earlier are most important in improving quality and preventing avoidable cost growth. It is a common saying that "if you've seen one integrated delivery system, you've seen one integrated delivery system." Yet it is likely that some elements are common across many IDSs and are more essential to success than others. It is also conceivable that some combination or critical mass of these and other elements needs to exist in order to ignite the flame of performance excellence that is the goal. At the moment no one knows what that critical mass of elements is.

Institutions engaged in Track A will want to identify benchmark organizations and learn from them in order to improve. As noted earlier, even successful multi-specialty group practices and integrated delivery systems vary in their mix of the key structural and process elements listed previously. Some of these organizations excel at some elements but not others. There is always room for the good to learn from the best.

Similarly, organizations moving along Track B will need to know which of many actions to take, and in what combination, in order to advance. One of the oft-stated reasons for the failure of many integrated delivery systems in the 1990s was that these nascent organizations had no real playbooks to follow in their development. Some succeeded and many failed as a result of management decisions that were frequently more intuitive than fact based. Therefore, more information is needed about what elements are essential and what really works. The best source of the needed information can be a critical self-examination by successful, large health care delivery organizations. The existing community of integrated delivery systems and large multispecialty group practices could do more, in combination with researchers and foundations such as The Commonwealth Fund, to accelerate the evolution of new knowledge in this area. For example, more needs to be known about the role that individual physician payment by salary versus FFS plays in promoting cost-conscious clinical decisions. Put another way, which matters more, the way a medical group is paid or the way it pays its physicians? There are other examples: To what extent can the EMR serve as a source of informal peer review within a medical group in the way that the earlier common paper chart used to? Are medical groups programming such transparency among providers into the systems they are buying and building? And how much directive decision support can be built into the EMR without creating physician resistance and reducing office productivity? Existing multispecialty group practices are well positioned to help answer these and similar questions.

Hospitals

View Physicians as Partners, not Competitors or Employees

As noted in several chapters, many physicians and hospital administrators come to work each day with quite different ideas about the appropriate role of the other. The traditional hospital board–professional medical staff model of governance—with dual lines of authority—was imperfect, but in the past it provided a rough script from which these players could act. But that model has begun to deteriorate. Partly in response to this deterioration, hospitals have begun to directly employ many more physicians in many more specialties than has been the case in the past. However, in some of these same communities, other physicians now choose to compete with hospitals through ambulatory care centers and small specialty hospitals. Thus, it would be natural for hospital administrators to view physicians either as competitors to be beaten or employees to be managed. Neither construct is likely to be a firm foundation for the success of either party in the long run.

There is an aspect of physician professionalism that chafes under institutional employment, especially when the physician feels disempowered yet still bears life-and-death responsibilities. This can lead physicians at best to passivity and underproductivity and at worst to disruptive behavior. There is a third construct possible—one in which hospital administrators and their boards reach out to staff physicians, employed or not, and create a governance model and an operational reality of partnership. In Chapter Five, Genovese describes some of the opportunities for operational improvements as a consequence of such improved mutual engagement. As Alexander and Young note in Chapter Seven, "Only through collaborative governance and joint decision making . . . will clinical care improve and efficiencies be achieved."

Support the Development and Success of Legitimate Physician Leaders

Medical schools rarely teach management and leadership skills. At Kaiser Permanente, we have traditionally tried to identify physicians with an interest and natural capabilities in these areas and then nurture them. Every clinical department chief is shown how to manage a budget, how to recruit and orient new physicians and employees, how to run a meeting, and how to manage individual and group performance. Physicians with broader institutional responsibilities are engaged in such disciplines as strategic planning, capital budgeting, marketing, and effective public speaking. These efforts are costly and time consuming but pay dividends many times over.

Smart partners make the best partners in an integrated system. It will be important for hospitals seeking to create robust integrated models to at least encourage, and at best directly support, physician leadership and management development.

Build a Business Case for Success with New Payment Models

Most U.S. hospitals are paid based on the amount of services provided, not the cost and quality of those services. Medicare payment by diagnosis-related groups (DRGs) and commercial payment by case rates create incentives to manage costs within a care episode but not incentives to manage the number of episodes (for example, admissions). Filled beds power the financial engine of most hospitals. But what happens if payers and physicians begin using forms of prepayment that include incentives to reduce hospital admissions and manage hospital costs, while current hospital financial incentives remain unchanged? Hospitals and physicians will be at odds. This is precisely the situation that has existed in the Medicare Physician Group Practice Demonstration project to date. Conversations with some of the involved medical group leaders suggest that the only reason that this conflict of financial interest has not been problematic is that the involved hospitals happen to have an undersupply of beds to meet the existing demand. Thus there are commercial patients available to fill beds left empty by better physician management of Medicare patients in ambulatory settings.

However, such a happy coincidence can't exist everywhere, as accountable care organizations involving physician-hospital integration become more widespread. In many geographical areas where beds are not undersupplied, hospitals will need financial incentives to participate in prepayment or shared savings models that are designed to reduce hospital admissions. Such an incentive environment exists in Kaiser Permanente and a few other fully integrated organizations. However, it is hard for most hospital administrators outside such entities to imagine a full bed as a cost entry on a budget rather than as a revenue entry.

As payers and policymakers grapple with the design and testing of new payment models, it would be beneficial for hospital leaders to be at the table, proposing options that would be advantageous to hospitals as well as physicians. For example, in the set of national reforms under consideration at the end of

2009, Congress had proposed an Innovation Center for the Medicare program, to pilot a variety of new payment models, and to encourage the formation of new delivery systems. When Medicare solicits projects for such an Innovation Center, hospitals could propose increases in payment for certain high-volume DRGs in proportion to and as a partial but substantive recompense for reduced unnecessary admissions for those DRGs. It would further be useful for such institutions to volunteer their hospitals as test environments for new payment models. This could be viewed as a natural extension of the goals of the American Hospital Association for clinical integration, as described in Chapter One.

Support the Formation of Multispecialty Group Practice

In the end, hospitals can choose to directly employ, compete with, or partner with the physicians in their communities. If they choose the latter, and a number of this book's authors argue they should, then they will want a competent, multifunctional and disciplined partner with which to work. The best examples of such, to date, are the nation's multispecialty group practices. (See Chapter Three for a description of these and other physician organizations and their relative strengths.) But there are currently not enough such groups; they are absent in some parts of the country; and, they are hard to build from the ground up. As described in Chapter Six, antitrust and other regulations currently inhibit hospitals from assisting independent physicians in many activities that would be part of multispecialty group practice formation. Assuming that well-crafted relief from some of these restrictions is part of delivery system reform efforts (for example, the Medicare Payment Advisory Commission has recommended such relief for gainsharing pilots[8]), hospitals should be ready to assist nascent multispecialty groups in their communities to form and grow in competency. Assuming a change in the regulatory environment, such support could begin with management and leadership training, as described earlier, and interim financial support for infrastructure development such as information technology systems. From such efforts will likely come future physician integration partners.

Payers, Plans, Employers, and Government as Payer

Support Payment Reforms That Move Away from Fee-for-Service

There is no more important point than this. Physician-hospital integration is an essential element in the development of health care organizations that can accept accountability for the cost and quality of health care services delivered to a community. This type of integration is unlikely to occur—and in fact has rarely occurred—in the environment of fee-for-service reimbursement. Many stakeholders now realize this to be true. The Massachusetts Special Commission on the Health Care Payment System, faced with rising health care costs after coverage expansion in that state, has set out to guide both public and private payers toward a variety of capitated or semicapitated models.[9] In Massachusetts and a few other states, local Blue Cross plans have begun to look for delivery system partners willing to try again with capitated models. On a national level, as previously noted, Congress may create a Medicare Innovation Center to pilot new payment models and encourage the formation of new delivery systems to receive those payments. (This center would be funded at one billion dollars a year for ten years, underscoring the importance Congress places on payment reform.)

Such activities should be encouraged and supported by payers both large and small. In particular, large employers engaged in self-funding health care services for their employees—typically under FFS reimbursement arrangements—should consider joining these payment reform activities. In many states, this will require changes in laws and regulations that specify fee-for-service payment to providers as a necessary characteristic of self-funded arrangements.

Experiment with Risk Sharing Rather Than Risk Transfer

There was a widespread retreat among payers from capitation in the mid-1990s (see Chapters Two and Four). This retreat was in sharp contrast to the enthusiasm for this model that had existed only a few years earlier. The change in payer attitude was partly due to the general public rejection of managed care and all restrictions associated with it. The change was also partly due to the frank failure of delivery systems, including established group practices and newly minted physician hospital organizations (PHOs), to successfully manage the transfer of financial risk. In many instances, providers lacked necessary cohesion and leadership to enable them successfully to accept and manage risk. In some cases, payers transferred too broad an array of risk, especially for nascent organizations to accept. For example, some medical groups accepted full-risk capitation that included pharmaceutical costs, with no control over health plan formularies and little experience in drug cost management. In other cases, the necessary management information systems were nonexistent. Although there were and still are examples of success with global capitation arrangements (for example, the California delegated model), these have been the exception, rather than the rule.

This negative experience with risk transfer appears to have so burned providers that when, as part of the 1997 Balanced Budget Act, Congress established a mechanism for global capitation in the Medicare Advantage Program (whose participants are known as *provider-sponsored organizations*), virtually no organizations applied, and the idea was effectively shelved. What seems to have been missed in this all too brief national foray into capitation is that such forms of prepayment do not need to involve complete risk transfer to be successful for both payer and provider.

Risk transfer has two dimensions: breadth and depth. *Breadth* refers to the number of elements of care delivery costs that are included under the payment (for example, primary care services, specialty referrals, hospital costs, pharmaceutical costs, and so on). *Depth* refers to how much of the costs, or how much of the cost variance from an established expenditure target, is transferred from the payer to the provider for a specific set of services. Kaiser Permanente has been very successful for decades with a risk transfer model that is very broad but modestly deep. The Permanente Medical Groups share financial responsibility with the health plan for all of the cost elements described earlier, but the year-end financial gain or loss of the group is limited by an established risk corridor. This corridor is set at a level that creates a group incentive to manage care appropriately but that is not so high as to require that the group establish significant financial reserves to cover expenses in the event of a loss. In essence, rather than complete risk *transfer*, Kaiser Permanente engages in risk *sharing* between payer and provider.

Such risk-sharing arrangements could be structured between provider organizations and both private and public payers. Both the breadth and depth of these arrangements could vary depending on the ability of the provider organization to manage risk, and could be advanced over time as the providers develop greater experience and competence in doing so. Federal or state government agencies could establish an interim stop-loss reinsurance system for developing capitation relationships, similar to that established by Congress during the implementation of Medicare Part D. The Massachusetts Special Commission on the Health Care Payment System intends to investigate the possibility of just such arrangements.[10]

Accept Reasonable Delivery System Consolidation

Some payers have been successful in capitated arrangements with integrated delivery systems. Still others are actively pursuing such new arrangements. On the other hand, some plans, large employers, and other purchasers are wary of any consolidation among physicians or between physician groups and hospitals. There is a fear that such integrated organizations will use their size to demand higher prices. This is not an unfounded concern. There are examples where just this dynamic has occurred. In some cases the Federal Trade Commission (FTC) has intervened; in other cases it has not.[11]

The transformations called for in this book will not take place without the support of commercial payers. Therefore it will be necessary to have processes in place to prevent the abusive exercise of market power. At the same time, it will also be necessary to *relax* some of the regulatory restrictions that make beneficial delivery system changes difficult (see Chapter Six). Protections against abuse of market power could include all-payer price regulation, clarification and *tightening* of some areas of antitrust enforcement, alternative dispute resolution related to payment levels, and state oversight of physician hospital organizations through state action exemption from federal antitrust regulation (see the following discussion). That said, it would be more productive for payers to engage in a dialogue about mitigating their legitimate concerns about market power than to seek to inhibit the development of integrated delivery systems entirely and thus lose for the nation the opportunity for the improvements in cost and quality that are possible in properly constructed delivery system reform.

Government as Lawmaker and Regulator

Mitigate Legal and Regulatory Obstacles to Integration

As mentioned earlier and well described in Chapter Six, there are a number of federal laws and regulations that either directly prohibit or create great uncertainty about the legality of certain physician-hospital activities. These include not only antitrust laws but also antikickback and self-referral laws, civil monetary penalties for withholding care from Medicare beneficiaries, and regulations regarding tax-exempt status. Each body of regulation serves a legitimate public interest. Yet, in practice, the totality of these laws and potential penalties has a chilling effect on innovations in delivery system structure and payment methodologies. Unless these barriers are addressed, progress toward physician-hospital integration as a key to delivery system reform will be inhibited.

It is possible that current health care reform will place the secretary of Health and Human Services (HHS) and her departments, including CMS, in the role of implementing many of the changes called for in the final legislation. This may well be the largest implementation challenge for a health secretary since the passage of the Medicare and Medicaid programs in the 1960s. There are at least two approaches that the secretary could take to address the regulatory problem. One approach is to serve as the convener of a group of regulators from different branches of government. The purpose of the group would be to mitigate the barriers to beneficial physician-hospital integration by voluntary changes to regulation or enforcement and to propose a set of legislative changes to allow the latitude needed for innovation.

Another approach is for the HHS secretary to propose, as part of the CMS Innovation Center, a series of CMS payment pilots that would contain the necessary regulatory exemptions. After several years, regulators could examine the behavioral dynamics within such pilots and begin to draw conclusions about what sort of regulatory changes could proceed without significant risk of fraud, abuse, quality compromise, or anticompetitive activities.

Alternatively, Congress could decide, as part of any follow-up health care reform clarification and extension legislation, to take a comprehensive new look at the regulatory environment. This would be a more delayed approach to the issue, but it may be inevitable if the escalation of health care expenditures continues unabated or, worse, accelerates.

Prevent Delivery System Monopolistic Pricing

As noted earlier, some purchasers of health care services have legitimate concerns about the potential for abusive pricing as a consequence of physician-hospital integration and the formation of accountable care organizations. Lawmakers, regulators, and enforcement agencies have a part to play, notwithstanding the needs described earlier, to help create an environment that allays those concerns.

One solution is to resolve this problem by explicit coordination of the expenditures of both private and public payers in an all-payer price regulation model. In addition, there are other potential methods that can be explored to prevent monopolistic pricing, short of all-payer rate regulation. As proposed earlier, federal regulatory agencies, such as the CMS Office of Inspector General, the Federal Trade Commission, and the Department of Justice, could form a special joint task force to review a number of the regulations referred to in Chapter Six. The agencies could then recommend a set of coordinated changes that would (1) make the formation of integrated delivery systems easier and (2) at the same time construct barriers to unacceptable pricing activities.

One market-based solution might be for payers and providers to enter into voluntary but binding arbitration agreements, using so-called baseball arbitration to resolve future disputes about payment levels. This is an idea suggested by John Bertko at the October 2009 meeting of the Medicare Payment Advisory Commission (MedPAC).[12] Baseball arbitration agreements bind the arbitrator to find entirely for one side of a dispute or another. There are no compromise judgments allowed. The impact of such a system is to moderate the behavior of both parties to an agreement, out of fear of being the loser in an arbitration judgment. It is conceivable that payer and provider entry into such agreements could be made a condition, by regulators, of certain safe harbors from regulatory scrutiny.

Another option would be for states to assume the role of watchdog for abusive market behavior by integrated providers through the use of state action exemptions from federal antitrust regulations. Such a solution requires that both the capacity and political will exist within a given state government to pursue this course.

Patients, Patient Advocates, and the Media

Understand the Value of Care Coordination; Expect Seamless Care

Payers, providers, and policymakers will never have much incentive to encourage physician-hospital integration if patients (voters) don't want it for themselves. But for the most part, patients do not understand the value of coordination of care, and they do not expect seamlessness among providers. Between 2007 and 2009, the Council of Accountable Physician Practices (CAPP), an affiliate of the American Medical Group Association, conducted a series of focus groups with consumers (patients) to test the common understanding of terminologies and concepts about the organization of health care delivery in this country. As described by Ross and colleagues, most patients were completely unfamiliar with words such as *coordinated care*, *multispecialty group practice*, and the like.[13] In subsequent focus groups, it took discussion of detailed case studies of uncoordinated care versus care properly coordinated across providers, settings, and time for the participants to grasp the difference. This phenomenon was particularly striking in parts of the country where integrated delivery systems had never existed. A fairly typical participant comment at the end of such a focus group was, "My goodness, where can I get that kind of wonderful care?"

During the extensive health care reform debate of 2009, several members of Congress commented in private to proponents of delivery system reform to this effect (paraphrasing): "These ideas are great. But they involve pretty big changes for people across the country, especially patients. We don't hear a call for what you are suggesting coming from our ordinary constituents. Until we do, how can such changes be expected to happen?"

These observations are indicators that the general case for integrated delivery systems has not been well made by their advocates. Within the geographical areas where established integrated delivery systems operate, their value is well understood and appreciated. But in areas of the country that lack such systems there is little understanding of their value. Despite efforts by the American Medical Group Association, the Council of Accountable Physician Practices, the Medical Group Management Association, and others, it has been difficult to overcome this public awareness challenge. Only recently, during the national discussion of delivery system reforms such as the medical home and accountable care organizations, has there begun to be media interest in these organizations. President Obama referred to the success of Kaiser Permanente, the Mayo Clinic, Geisinger Health System, and the Cleveland Clinic on several occasions during the health care reform discussions in the summer and fall of 2009.

There is an opportunity for patient advocates, such as the American Association of Retired Persons (AARP), Families USA, and members of the health care media to engage constituents and the public in a discussion of the pros and cons of various delivery system organizational models. This has begun already, through the efforts of popular, mainstream (as opposed to academic) authors such as Shannon Brownlee and Dr. Atul Gawande.[14] But more remains to be done. During the later stages of the health reform debate in 2009, it became clear that many more people understood the ins and outs of the public plan option than had even a basic understanding of the potential impact of delivery system changes.

Kaiser Permanente and other integrated delivery system strive to provide patients with seamless care. That means that handoffs from primary care physician to specialty physician and from office to hospital and back again and the management of myriad services for patients with complex conditions are coordinated by the system itself, and not by an ill, sometimes confused, and often anxious patient. No organization can be perfect at such a task, but far too many patients in the United States today are bouncing from one physician to another, one institution to another, and don't receive the rudiments of care coordination that can and should be within the reach of every American. More efforts to tell this story are needed.

Finally, patients are often poorly informed about the likely impact of changes in the way their health plans pay their doctors. Payment of group practices by capitation rather than fee-for-service and payment of individual physicians by salary rather than fee-for-service create different incentives for physicians. Many informed observers, including the former editor of the *New England Journal of Medicine*, are currently advocating (again) for movement from the former to the latter in each case.[15] Some patients and patient advocates have strong feelings about such a transition. More public understanding of the proper relationship between payment modes and the ideal environment for a high-quality, ethical practice, worthy of patient trust, is needed and should be welcomed.

Conclusion

As this book went to press, the nation was poised on the first step of an ascent toward a fairer, more inclusive health care system and, it is to be hoped, toward one that produces better value for its citizens. It is likely that expansion of coverage will prove to be easier than bending the cost curve to help produce that higher value. Health care is one-sixth of the U.S. economy, a sum larger than the gross domestic products of all but a few nations. It has its own interests and momentum, fueled by technological advances that often produce real value but sometimes only increase costs.

Most health care costs derive from the judgments and actions of physicians and often are expended within the walls of the nation's hospitals. Incremental efforts over the last two decades to slow the growth of health care professional and institutional costs have had only small effects. What is needed is a fundamental change in the structure of health care delivery, and the creation of payment systems that reward quality and appropriateness of care, not volume of services. We need a system in which physicians and hospitals, the two principal health care agents of the public trust, work together in a cooperative environment designed to serve the needs of all Americans for both high-quality services and affordability. This change needs to happen now, not only to help the nation recover its financial strength but also so that we may pass down a sound health care system to meet the future needs of our children and our grandchildren. We, the editors and authors of this book, hope that the information we have imparted here will help us all along that path.

Notes

1. The Commonwealth Fund Commission on a High Performance Health System, *Framework for a High Performance Health System for the United States*" (New York: The Commonwealth Fund, 2006), http://www.commonwealthfund.org/Content/Publications/Fund-Reports/2006/Aug/Framework-for-a-High-Performance-Health-System-for-the-United-States.aspx.
2. Physicians participating in FFS Medicare receive annual per-service-unit increases or decreases in payment based on a formula commonly known as the Sustainable Growth Rate (SGR) formula. In basic terms, the formula raises payment rates in response to GDP increases and lowers rate in response to per beneficiary increases in service volume. Because service volume has overwhelmed GDP increases in recent years, the SGR formula has called for "negative increases" (in other words, decreases). Congress has overridden the formula repeatedly, generally keeping physician payment rates close to flat. As this book went to press, Congress was considering repealing the SGR formula.
3. Business Wire, "Blue Cross Blue Shield of Massachusetts Signs First Groups to Its Alternative Quality Contract," January 14, 2009, http://www.thefreelibrary.com/Blue+Cross+Blue+Shield+of+Massachusetts+Signs+First+Groups+to+Its+New . . . -a0191988260 (accessed October 20, 2009).
4. D. Berwick, "A User's Manual for the IOM's 'Quality Chasm' Report," *Health Affairs* 21, no. 3 (2002): 80–90; B. James, "Quality Improvement Opportunities in Health Care: Making It Easy to Do It Right," *Journal of Managed Care Pharmacy* 8, no. 5 (2002): 394–99.

5. A. B. Haynes and others, "A Surgical Quality Checklist to Reduce Morbidity and Mortality in a Global Population," *New England Journal of Medicine* 30, no. 5 (2009): 491–99.

6. Centers for Medicare and Medicaid Services, "Physician Groups Earn Payments for Improving the Quality of Care for Patients with Chronic Disease" (press release), August 14, 2004, http://www.cms.hhs.gov/apps/media/press/release.asp?Counter=3239; R. Gillies, K. Chenok, S. Shortell, G. Pawlson, and others, "The Impact of Health Plan Delivery System Organization on Clinical Quality and Patient Satisfaction," *Health Services Research* 41, no. 4, pt. 1 (2006), 1181–99.

7. L. Casalino, R. R. Gillies, S. M. Shortell, J. A. Schmittdiel, and others, "External Incentives, Information Technology, and Organized Processes to Improve Health Care Quality for Patients with Chronic Diseases," *JAMA* 289, no. 4 (2003): 434–41.

8. Medicare Payment Advisory Commission, "Physician Owned Specialty Hospitals" (statement of Glenn M. Hackbarth, JD, before the Subcommittee on Health of the Committee on Ways and Means, U.S. House of Representatives, March 8, 2005), http://www.medpac.gov/publications/congressional_testimony/030805_TestimonySpecHosp-Sen.pdf.

9. Commonwealth of Massachusetts, Division of Health Care Financing and Policy, "Recommendations of the Special Commission on the Health Care Payment System" (July 16, 2009), www.mass.gov/Eeohhs2/docs/dhcfp/pc/Final_Report/Final_Report.pdf.

10. Commonwealth of Massachusetts, "Recommendations of the Special Commission."

11. Federal Trade Commission, "FTC Challenges Carilion's Acquisition of Outpatient Medical Clinics" (press release), July 24, 2009, http://www.ftc.gov/opa/2009/07/carilion.shtm.

12. Medicare Payment Advisory Commission, "Transcript of Public Meeting on Oct. 9, 2009,"http://www.medpac.gov/transcripts/1008-1009MedPAC.final.pdf (accessed October 21, 2009).

13. M. Ross and others, "From Our Lips to Whose Ears: Consumer Reaction to Our Current Health Care Dialect," *Permanente Journal* 13, no. 1 (2009): 8–16.

14. S. Brownlee, *Overtreated: Why Too Much Medicine Is Making Us Sicker and Poorer* (New York: Bloomsbury USA, 2007); A. Gawande, "The Cost Conundrum: What a Texas Town Can Teach Us About Health Care," *New Yorker*, June 1, 2009, 36–44.

15. A. Relman, "Doctors as the Key to Health Care Reform," *New England Journal of Medicine* 361, no. 14 (2009): 1225–29.

INDEX